Pulmonary and Respiratory Diseases and Disorders

nova
Medicine & Health
New York

Pulmonary and Respiratory Diseases and Disorders

Understanding and Treating Acute Pulmonary Embolism
James K. Edwards (Editor)
2022. ISBN: 979-8-88697-149-1 (Softcover)
2022. ISBN: 979-8-88697-398-3 (eBook)

Chronic Obstructive Pulmonary Disease: From Diagnosis to Treatment
Jaber S. Alqahtani, PhD (Editor)
2022. ISBN: 979-8-88697-333-4 (Hardcover)
2022. ISBN: 979-8-88697-396-9 (eBook)

Interstitial Lung Disease: From Diagnosis to Treatment
Roberto G. Carbone, MD, FCCP (Editor)
Francesco Puppo, MD (Editor)
Keith Wille, MD, MSPH (Editor)
Pallav Shah, MD (Editor)
2022. ISBN: 978-1-68507-926-0 (Hardcover)
2022. ISBN: 979-8-88697-068-5 (eBook)

A Clinical Manual of Sarcoidosis
Vikas Pathak, MD (Editor)
Shambhu Aryal, MD (Editor)
2022. ISBN: 978-1-68507-681-8 (Hardcover)
2022. ISBN: 978-1-68507-782-2 (eBook)

Pulmonary Vascular Disorders
Francesco Puppo, MD (Editor),
Roberto G. Carbone, MD, FCCP (Editor),
Victor F. Tapson, MD, FCCP, FRCP (Editor)
2021. ISBN: 978-1-53619-458-6 (Hardcover)
2021. ISBN: 978-1-53619-553-8 (eBook)

More information about this series can be found at
https://novapublishers.com/product-category/series/pulmonary-and-respiratory-diseases-and-disorders/

Antonio M. Esquinas
Editor

Ventilator Induced Lung Injury in Non-Invasive Ventilatory Support

Pathophysiology, Treatment and Prevention

nova
Medicine & Health
New York

DOI: https://doi.org/10.52305/CNAO0121.

NOTICE TO THE READER

Library of Congress Cataloging-in-Publication Data

Names: Esquinas, Antonio M., editor.
Title: Ventilator induced lung injury in non-invasive ventilatory support : pathophysiology, treatment and prevention / editor, Antonio M. Esquinas, MD, PHD, FCCP, FAARC, Intensive Care Unit Hospital Morales Meseguer, Murcia, Spain; Director, International School of Non-Invasive Ventilation; Director, International Non Invasive Ventilation Expert of College.
Description: New York : Nova Science Publishers, [2023] | Series: Pulmonary and respiratory diseases and disorders | Includes bibliographical references and index. |
Identifiers: LCCN 2023021922 (print) | LCCN 2023021923 (ebook) | ISBN 9798886978407 (hardcover) | ISBN 9798886978872 (adobe pdf)
Subjects: LCSH: Respirators (Medical equipment) | Respiratory insufficiency--Equipment and supplies. | Lungs--Wounds and injuries--Equipment and supplies. | Artificial respiration--Equipment and supplies.
Classification: LCC RC735.I5 V44 2023 (print) | LCC RC735.I5 (ebook) | DDC 616.20028/4--dc23/eng/20230606
LC record available at https://lccn.loc.gov/2023021922
LC ebook record available at https://lccn.loc.gov/2023021923

Published by Nova Science Publishers, Inc. † New York

To our patients, our major motivation.

To my wife and daughters.

Contents

Preface

Over the last two decades, it has been demonstrated that the use of non-invasive mechanical ventilation systems, in their various non-invasive, positive or negative options, as well as nasal high-flow, has proven to be very useful in various clinical indications. However, one essential aspect of all medical treatment is to determine how non-invasive ventilatory support can be a determinant of ventilatory-induced lung injury. While this concept and observation classically comes from experimental and clinical observations in patients with invasive mechanical ventilation and acute respiratory distress syndrome, there are observations and possible mechanisms that can be observed when applying non-invasive ventilatory support options. This book analyses the pathophysiology mechanisms that relate to this process commonly referred to as patient self-inflicted lung injury.

The book is structured on the description of these mechanisms (atelectrauma, barotrauma, biotrauma, volutrauma and atelectrauma, hyperoxemia, etc.), lung mechanics and inflammatory response, description of dyspnea in spontaneous acute lung injury, and pathophysiology.

An analysis of the time course of ventilator-induced lung injury in patients with non-invasive ventilation is performed, based on an analysis of summary animal studies and clinical implications. Lastly, this book provides recommendations on diagnosis and prevention based on an analysis of the monitoring of pressure/volume curves and flow waveforms.

We consider that an exhaustive knowledge of the pathophysiology is essential during all the options of non-invasive ventilatory support, interpretation of the concept of a patient self-induced lung injury in the most common scenarios of use and open to future editions the new forms of diagnosis and prevention of these situations.

One cannot consider such a commonly used technique without knowing the pathophysiology of those determinants that can limit a successful application of the technique.

"There will be no excellence in your treatment...
if we do not know the essence of its mechanism."

Antonio M. Esquinas MD, PhD,
Murcia, Spain,
November 3, 2022

Chapter 1

Epidemiology

Inês Teixeira Farinha*, MD
Pulmonology Department,
Coimbra Hospital and University Centre, Coimbra, Portugal

Abstract

Ventilator-induced lung injury is the acute lung injury inflicted or aggravated by positive-pressure ventilation during treatment, occurring both in invasive as well as non-invasive ventilation.

Four main mechanisms of VILI will be described: alveolar inspiratory and/or expiratory stress inducing overdistension (volutrauma), interfaces between collapsed or edema-filled alveoli and surrounding open alveoli, acting as stress raisers (barotrauma), alveoli that continuously open and close with tidal breathing (atelectotrauma), and systemic inflammatory response (biotrauma).

Mechanical ventilation potentially injures both normal and diseased lungs; however, the injury is much more severe in the latter. It is important to be able to recognize VILI to prevent the progression of lung damage.

Keywords: ventilator-induced lung injury, non-invasive ventilation, respiratory insufficiency

Introduction

The emergence of positive-pressure ventilation dates back to the 1950s polio outbreak [1]. The experience obtained from this epidemic became the

* Corresponding Author's Email: i.t.farinha@gmail.com.

In: Ventilator Induced Lung Injury in Non-Invasive Ventilatory Support
Editor: Antonio M. Esquinas
ISBN: 979-8-88697-840-7

foundation of critical care practice. Over more than 7 decades, positive-pressure ventilation devices have significantly evolved in both pediatric and adult patients and can now be delivered without intubation, referred to as non-invasive ventilation (NIV) [2]. There is currently robust evidence documenting its efficacy in altering outcomes in chronic obstructive pulmonary disease, cardiogenic pulmonary edema, acute respiratory failure in COVID-19 patients, and acute respiratory failure in immunocompromised patients [3]. However, despite being a beneficial intervention, positive-pressure ventilation must be carefully titrated since it may be associated with lung damage and lead to ventilator-induced lung injury (VILI) [4].

VILI is the acute lung injury inflicted or aggravated by positive-pressure ventilation during treatment [5]. It can occur during invasive as well as NIV and proven to contribute to mortality in patients with acute respiratory distress syndrome (ARDS) and might contribute significantly to the morbidity and mortality of other critically ill patients [6]. Though mechanical ventilation potentially injures both normal and diseased lungs, the injury will be much more severe in the latter due to higher microscale stresses [5]. Despite being used interchangeably, the term 'ventilator-associated lung injury' (VALI) refers to the presence of lung injury during mechanical ventilation when a causal link is not ascertained [7].

The notion of injury by mechanical ventilation was first described in the mid-18th century by John Fothergill [8, 9]. He postulated that mouth-to-mouth ventilation might be a better option than machine bellows in resuscitation since "the lungs of one man may bear, without injury, as great a force as those of another man can exert, which by the bellows cannot always be determined" [8]. During the 1952 polio epidemic, structural lung damages caused by mechanical ventilation were documented [10]. Thereafter, in 1967, the term "respirator lung" used to describe the postmortem lung injury on autopsy of patients exposed to positive-pressure ventilation and whose lungs showed extensive alveolar infiltrates and hyaline membrane formation [5]. Over the past decades, evidence on VILI mechanisms and etiology has evolved, which contributed to new lines of investigation towards personalizing lung-protective strategies [11].

Classically, four mechanisms of VILI have described, which include: alveolar inspiratory and/or expiratory stress inducing overdistension (volutrauma), interfaces between collapsed or edema-filled alveoli and surrounding open alveoli, acting as stress raisers (barotrauma), alveoli that continuously open and close with tidal breathing (atelectotrauma), and systemic inflammatory response (biotrauma) [7,12-16]. Other mechanisms, which are currently studies, may include heterogeneous local lung mechanics, alveolar stress frequency, and stress failure of pulmonary capillaries [4]. Furthermore, variation in the expression of genetically determined inflammatory mediators has shown to affect VILI susceptibility [17]. It is important to be able to recognize and manage VILI to improve gas exchange and prevent the progression of lung damage, especially in the presence of significant lung disease.

The incidence of VILI is still unclear, both in adult and pediatric patients. However, in the adult population, this injury expected to be more frequent in ARDS patients receiving mechanical ventilation [5,18]. When the lungs injured, mechanical ventilation will further damage them, in the absence of lung-protective strategies [5]. A study conducted on 332 mechanically ventilated patients without acute lung injury at the beginning of ventilation found the development of VILI in 24% of patients within the first five days [19].

Conclusion

Barotrauma has been employed in studies as a surrogate measure of VALI, because it has a specific radiologic and clinical definition. However, its relationship to the microstructural lesions of VALI is unknown [19]. The incidence of barotrauma in patients with ARDS has decreased markedly in recent years due to changes in the approach to mechanical ventilation, with reduction of tidal volume and the use of lower plateau pressures. Prospective ARDS studies report an incidence of barotrauma ranging from 5-10% (in meta-analyses) and from 5-6% (in clinical trials) [20-22]. No geographic influences are known to affect the incidence of barotrauma. Age, sex, or ethnicity not expected to influence barotrauma. However, it is known that lung compliance tends to decrease with age, which may play a role in the risk for barotrauma in older patients [23].

References

[1] Ibsen B. The anaesthetist's viewpoint on the treatment of respiratory complications in poliomyelitis during the epidemic in Copenhagen, 1952. *Proc. R Soc. Med.* 1954; 47(1):72-4.

[2] MacIntyre N. Design Features of Modern Mechanical Ventilators. *Clin. Chest Med.* 2016;37(4):607-13.

[3] Pierson D J. History and epidemiology of noninvasive ventilation in the acute-care setting. *Respir. Care.* 2009;54(1):40-52.

[4] Katira BH. Ventilator-Induced Lung Injury: Classic and Novel Concepts. *Respir. Care.* 2019;64(6):629-37.

[5] Anjum A K A F. *Ventilator-Induced Lung Injury* (VILI). 2021.

[6] Brower R G, Matthay M A, Morris A, Schoenfeld D, Thompson BT, Wheeler A. Ventilation with lower tidal volumes as compared with traditional tidal volumes for acute lung injury and the acute respiratory distress syndrome. *N. Engl. J. Med.* 2000;342(18):1301-8.

[7] Cruz FF, Ball L, Rocco P R M, Pelosi P. Ventilator-induced lung injury during controlled ventilation in patients with acute respiratory distress syndrome: less is probably better. *Expert Rev. Respir. Med.* 2018;12(5):403-14.

[8] Fothergill J. XI. Observations on a case published in the last volume of the medical essays, &c. of recovering a man dead in appearance, by distending the lungs with air. Printed at Edinburgh, 1744; by John Fothergill, Licent. *Coll. Med. Lond.* Philosophical Transactions of the Royal Society of London. 1744;43(475):275-81.

[9] Slutsky A S. History of Mechanical Ventilation. From Vesalius to Ventilator-induced Lung Injury. *Am. J. Respir. Crit. Care Med.* 2015;191(10):1106-15.

[10] Avignon P D, Hedenstrom G, Hedman C. Pulmonary complications in respirator patients. *Acta Med. Scand. Suppl.* 1956;316:86-90.

[11] Tremblay LN, Slutsky AS. Ventilator-induced lung injury: from the bench to the bedside. *Intensive Care Med*. 2006;32(1):24-33.

[12] Chen L, Xia HF, Shang Y, Yao SL. Molecular Mechanisms of Ventilator-Induced Lung Injury. *Chin. Med. J.* (Engl). 2018;131(10):1225-31.

[13] Curley GF, Laffey JG, Zhang H, Slutsky AS. Biotrauma and Ventilator-Induced Lung Injury: Clinical Implications. *Chest.* 2016;150(5):1109-17.

[14] Luciano Gattinoni· John J Marini· Francesca Collino· Giorgia Maiolo, Francesca Rapetti, Tommaso Tonetti, Francesco Vasques· Michael Quintel. The future of mechanical ventilation: lessons from the present and the past. *Crit. Care.* 2017;21(1): 183.

[15] Slutsky AS, Ranieri VM. Ventilator-induced lung injury. *N. Engl. J. Med.* 2013;369(22):2126-36.

[16] Wang Z Y, Li T, Wang C T, Xu L, Gao X J. Assessment of 1-year Outcomes in Survivors of Severe Acute Respiratory Distress Syndrome Receiving Extracorporeal Membrane Oxygenation or Mechanical Ventilation: A Prospective Observational Study. *Chin. Med. J.* (Engl). 2017;130(10):1161-8.

[17] Sang-Bum Hong· Yong Huang, Liliana Moreno-Vinasco, Saad Sammani, Jaideep Moitra, Joseph W Barnard, Shwu-Fan Ma, Tamara Mirzapoiazova, Carrie Evenoski, Ryan R Reeves, Eddie T Chiang, Gabriel D Lang, Aliya N Husain, Steven M Dudek, Jeffrey R Jacobson, Shui Q Ye, Yves A Lussier, Joe G N Garcia. Essential role of pre-B-cell colony enhancing factor in ventilator-induced lung injury. *Am. J. Respir. Crit. Care Med.* 2008;178(6):605-17.

[18] Piastra M, Conti G. Ventilator-induced lung injury in childhood. Minerva Anestesiol. 2018;84(5):543-5.

[19] International consensus conferences in intensive care medicine: Ventilator-associated Lung Injury in ARDS. This official conference report was cosponsored by the American Thoracic Society, The European Society of Intensive Care Medicine, and The Societé de Réanimation de Langue Française, and was approved by the ATS Board of Directors, July 1999. *Am. J. Respir. Crit. Care Med.* 1999;160(6):2118-24.

[20] Matthias Briel· Maureen Meade, Alain Mercat, Roy G Brower, Daniel Talmor, Stephen D Walter, Arthur S Slutsky, Eleanor Pullenayegum, Qi Zhou, Deborah Cook, Laurent Brochard, Jean-Christophe M Richard, Francois Lamontagne, Neera Bhatnagar, Thomas E Stewart, Gordon Guyatt. Higher vs lower positive end-expiratory pressure in patients with acute lung injury and acute respiratory distress syndrome: systematic review and meta-analysis. *Jama.* 2010;303(9):865-73.

[21] Claude Guérin, Jean Reignier, Jean-Christophe Richard, Pascal Beuret, Arnaud Gacouin, Thierry Boulain, Emmanuelle Mercier, Michel Badet, Alain Mercat, Olivier Baudin, Marc Clavel, Delphine Chatellier, Samir Jaber, Sylvène Rosselli, Jordi Mancebo, Michel Sirodot, Gilles Hilbert, Christian Bengler, Jack Richecoeur, Marc Gainnier, Frédérique Bayle, Gael Bourdin, Véronique Leray, Raphaele Girard, Loredana Baboi, Louis Ayzac Prone positioning in severe acute respiratory distress syndrome. *N. Engl. J. Med.* 2013;368(23):2159-68.

[22] Claude Guérin· Jean Reignier, Jean-Christophe Richard, Pascal Beuret, Arnaud Gacouin, Thierry Boulain, Emmanuelle Mercier, Michel Badet, Alain Mercat, Olivier Baudin, Marc Clavel, Delphine Chatellier, Samir Jaber, Sylvène Rosselli, Jordi Mancebo, Michel Sirodot, Gilles Hilbert, Christian Bengler, Jack Richecoeur, Marc Gainnier, Frédérique Bayle, Gael Bourdin, Véronique Leray, Raphaele Girard, Loredana Baboi, Louis Ayzac, PROSEVA Study Group. Neuromuscular blockers in early acute respiratory distress syndrome. *N. Engl. J. Med.* 2010;363(12):1107-16.

[23] Antonio Anzueto· Fernando Frutos-Vivar, Andres Esteban, Inmaculada Alía, Laurent Brochard, Thomas Stewart, Salvador Benito, Martin J Tobin, Jose Elizalde, Fernando Palizas, Cide M David, Jorge Pimentel, Marco González, Luis Soto, Gabriel D'Empaire, Paolo Pelosi. Incidence, risk factors and outcome of barotrauma in mechanically ventilated patients. *Intensive Care Med.* 2004;30(4):612-9.

Chapter 2

Dyspnea in Spontaneous Acute Lung Injury: Pathophysiology

Catarina Carvalho Cordes Amaral Barata*, **MD**
West Lisbon Hospital Center, Lisboa, Portugal

Abstract

Acute lung injury (ALI) and acute respiratory distress syndrome (ARDS) represent spectrums of a complex process of progressive respiratory failure, leading to low alveolar ventilation/perfusion ratios (VA/Q), and abnormal shunting of O_2, loss of control of vascular ton, and right ventricular failure. Clinically it may present with dyspnea, a subjective awareness of the sensation of uncomfortable breathing, that results from a mismatch between afferent receptors and central respiratory motor activity and a dissociation between pulmonary ventilation and respiratory drive. Multiple factors in lung ventilation influence the appearance and intensity dyspnea, through activation of mechanoreceptors int the lung, airways and chest wall and chemoreceptors in the carotid bodies and through exaggerated ventilatory response.

Keywords: acute respiratory distress syndrome, acute lung injury, dyspnea, hypoxemia, ventilation-perfusion mismatch

Introduction

Acute lung injury (ALI) and acute respiratory distress syndrome (ARDS) represent spectrums of a complex process of progressive respiratory failure,

* Corresponding Author's Email: catarinabarata22@gmail.com.

In: Ventilator Induced Lung Injury in Non-Invasive Ventilatory Support
Editor: Antonio M. Esquinas
ISBN: 979-8-88697-840-7

characterized by rapid onset, diffuse, bilateral alveolar damage, capillary leakage and protein rich pulmonary oedema leading to low alveolar ventilation/perfusion ratios (VA/Q), and abnormal shunting of O_2. Clinically it is characterized by dyspnea, tachypnea and cyanosis refractory to oxygen therapy, and on chest X-ray it shows diffuse alveolar infiltrates with non-cardiogenic pulmonary edema. ALI can be caused by multiple mechanisms, including pulmonary and extra-pulmonary illness. The most frequent causes are pulmonary-specific: pneumonia, aspiration, pulmonary embolism, chest trauma or inhaled noxious gases. Systemic conditions include sepsis, burns, massive transfusions, pancreatitis and hemorrhagic shock [1, 2].

Clinical Definition of ALI/ARDS

Since its first description by Ashbaugh *et al.* [3] in 1967, the definition of ALI/ARDS has undergone several changes. The updated and revised Berlin definition for ALI/ARDS [4] is an approach of combining consensus discussions with empirical evaluation in order to standardize and validate this syndrome, recognized as a major clinical problem worldwide. Table 1 shows Berlin criteria for acute respiratory distress syndrome.

Table 1. Berlin criteria for acute respiratory distress syndrome

Onset	Within 1 week of a known clinical insult or new or worsening respiratory symptoms.
Oxygenation	Mild ARDS: $PaO_2/FiO_2 > 200mmHg \leq 300mmHg$. Moderate ARDS: $PaO_2/FiO_2 > 100mmHg \leq 200mmHg$. Severe ARDS $PaO_2/FiO_2 \leq 100mmHg$.
PEEP	Minimum $5cmH_20$ PEEP by invasive mechanical ventilation or noninvasive ventilation.
Chest imaging	Bilateral opacities not fully explained by effusions, lung collapse or nodules on chest X-ray or CT.
Origin of oedema	Respiratoy failure not fully explained by cardiac failure of fluid overload (echocardiography excluding hydrostatic oedema if no risk factor present).

Abbreviations: PEEP: positive end-expiratory pressure; PaO_2: arterial oxygen tension; FiO_2: inspiratory oxygen fraction; CT: computed tomography.

Pathophysiology of ALI/ARDS

Acute lung injury processes through several phases after an injury. The acute, exudative phase (up to 7 days) is characterized by rapid onset of respiratory dysfunction. In this phase there is activation of alveolar macrophages, neutrophils, platelets, and epithelial cells, which secrete inflammatory mediators and cells, leading to increased vascular permeability through destruction of epithelial-endothelial barrier and leak of protein-rich fluid and blood cells into the interstitium and alveoli. These changes result in damage of surfactant-producing alveolar type II cells with surfactant loss, formation of hyaline membranes, alveolar atelectasis and hemorrhage, pulmonary oedema, and decreased lung compliance [5, 6]. Alveolar vascular damage also leads to altered vasomotor tone (vasoconstriction and vasodilation) and formation of microthrombi. This results in pulmonary hypertension with increasing right ventricular afterload and ventricular dysfunction. Combined endothelial and epithelial damage ends up with worsening ventilation-perfusion mismatch, loss of hypoxic pulmonary vasoconstriction and refractory hypoxia [7, 8].

The proliferative phase takes two to three weeks and initiates the repair process of the lung. Anti-inflammatory cytokines and cells deactivate neutrophils and macrophages; type II alveolar cells proliferate and establish the epithelial lining and surfactant production.

The excess fluid in the alveoli and interstitium is drawn by re-expressed alveolar ion channels and aquaporins and the endothelial cells reestablish vascular integrity [6, 7].

The fibrotic phase, only occur in some patients with ongoing inflammation and persistent endothelial and epithelial damage and is associated with increased morbidity and mortality [7].

Clinical Presentation in ALI/ARDS

In ALI/ARDS most patients follow similar clinical courses. Patients typically present with dyspnea, hypoxemia and cyanosis. On examination patients may have tachypnea, tachycardia, diffuse crackles over the chest, increased work of breathing, and use of accessory respiratory muscles. Laboratory changes are nonspecific and include leukocytosis, evidence of disseminated intravascular coagulation, and lactic acidosis. Blood gases may show severe hypoxemia, decreased PaO2/FiO2, and acute respiratory acidosis. On the chest X-ray, interstitial pulmonary oedema with bilateral diffuse infiltrates may be identified [8].

Dyspnea in ALI/ARDS

Dyspnea, also known as shortness of breath, is a subjective awareness of the sensation of uncomfortable breathing. Dyspnea begins with a physiological impairment (either respiratory, cardiovascular or metabolic derangements) that stimulates pulmonary and extrapulmonary afferent receptors, which are responsible for the transmission of the information to the cerebral cortex, where the sensation of discomfort (increased respiratory work/effort, tightness, or air hunger) is perceived.

The mismatch between afferent receptors and central respiratory motor activity leads to a dissociation between pulmonary ventilation and respiratory drive [9].

Several afferent pathways are responsible for the perception of breathlessness: Atelectasis and pulmonary oedema activates juxta capillary receptors; bronchoconstriction signal stretch receptors in the lung; and the tension on respiratory muscles activates muscle spindles in the chest wall; the metabolic derangements stimulate the chemoreceptors in the carotid bodies and medulla, which stimulate breathing by changing the sensitivity of central chemoreceptors.

The efferent signals are the motor neuronal signals that send information to the respiratory muscles [9, 10].

Dyspnea occurs when there is an increase above usual levels of afferent information from the peripheral sensors and the central neural output does not produce the expected result of motor commands to the ventilatory muscles (airflow or ventilation).

The extent of the mismatch of this information determines the intensity of dyspnea. The sensory cortex is simultaneously activated when motor signals are sent to the chest wall, resulting in the conscious sensation of muscular effort and breathlessness [10, 11].

In ALI/ARDS several changes in lung ventilation influence the appearance of dyspnea:

1) *VA/Q mismatch and physiological shunting*: In ARDS, atelectasis, pulmonary oedema, and air space consolidation, results in increased

dead space and shunt, where a lung unit is not ventilated and perfusion is preserved. In severe cases of ARDS, the shunt area may exced 50% of the lung, leading to severe hypoxemia. Also the diffusion between capillaries and alveoli may be affected: the fluid in the lungs increases the effective thickness of the alveolar wall and decreases the area of gas exchange, resulting in perfusion without ventilation and shunting, leading to hypoxemia and hypercapnia [12].

2) *Decreased lung compliance*: The alveolar epithelium destruction and alveolar flooding leads to surfactant loss, increased surface tension and alveolar atelectasis during end-expiration, which fail to expand during inspiration due to high alveolar opening pressures. This results in decreased lung compliance, which, in turn, originates rapid, shallow breathing, and reduced functional residual capacity, aggravating dyspnea [13].
3) *Pulmonary hypertension and right ventricular failure*: Activation of pulmonary microvascular endothelium leads to imbalance between vasodilating and vasoconstricting mediators and a shift to a prothrombotic phenotype. It results in capillary and larger pulmonary arteries, veins, and lymphatics occlusion due to thromboemboli and fibrinous obliteration. A loss of control of vascular tone, with an excess of pulmonary vasoconstrictor over vasodilator substances increases vascular tone, leading to acute rises in pulmonary vascular resistance, and later, to vascular remodeling, with increased thickness of the pulmonary arterial smooth muscle layer, and neomuscularization of previously non muscularized vessels. These pathological factors contribute to VA/Q mismatch and right ventricular dysfunction. This also result in hypoxemia, which stimulates chemoreceptors in the carotid bodies and medulla [13].

These conditions together will activate the mechanoreceptors in the lungs, airways and chest wall and the chemoreceptors in the carotid bodies and medullae.

However, the response to this afferent information may be compromised due to exaggerated ventilatory response in the brain (secondary to systemic inflammation and organ dysfunction, acidosis and shock) and to increased respiratory load and muscle weakness. The consequence is a rapid shallow breathing with increased respiratory rate but decreased tidal volume. This mismatch of information and deranged response determines the emergence and intensity of dyspnea [14].

Treatment of Dyspnea

Opioids have been the most widely studied drug in the treatment of dyspnea in patients with a variety of conditions. However, evidence of long-term efficacy is limited and conflicting. In addition, opioids are associated with several adverse effects [9]. The treatment of dyspnea involves treating the underlying pathology. In the case of ARDS, it will include oxygen therapy, non-invasive ventilation, or even invasive mechanical ventilation in the more severe cases, antibiotic therapy, corticosteroid therapy and sedation when necessary, and other treatments aimed at the initial insult that triggered the ARDS.

Conclusion

Acute lung injury and acute respiratory distress syndrome represent two spectrums of a complex process of progressive respiratory failure, and it is a major clinical problem worldwide. It is characterized by rapid onset, diffuse, bilateral alveolar damage, capillary leakage and protein rich pulmonary oedema. Acute lung injury processes through several phases after an injury: the exudative phase, the proliferative phase and the fibrotic phase where there is activation of multiple inflammatory mediators and cells leading to alveolar damage and atelectasis, pulmonary oedema, altered vasomotor tone, decreased lung compliance formation of microthrombi and right ventricular dysfunction and ultimately leading to severe respiratory dysfunction.

Dyspnea, also known as shortness of breath, is a subjective awareness of the sensation of uncomfortable breathing and is a common symptom in ARDS. It occurs when there is an increase above usual levels of afferent information from the peripheral sensors and the central neural output does not produce the expected result of motor commands to the ventilatory muscles (airflow or ventilation). The extent of the mismatch of this information determines the intensity of dyspnea.

Multiple factors in ARDS influence the appearance of dyspnea: VA/Q mismatch and physiological shunting, impaired diffusion, decreased lung compliance, microthrombi formation, pulmonary hypertension and right ventricular failure, and the exaggerated ventilatory response in the brain due to systemic inflammation, organ dysfunction, acidosis and shock. The treatment of dyspnea involves treating the underlying pathology. In the case of ARDS, it will include oxygen therapy, non-invasive ventilation, or even invasive mechanical ventilation in the more severe cases and other targeted therapies. Opioids use is limited and conflicting.

References

[1] Dushianthan A, Grocott MPW, Postle AD and Cusack R. 2011. "Acute Respiratory Distress Syndrome and Acute Lung Injury." *Postgraduate Medical Journal,* 87 (1031): 612-22. https://doi.org/10.1136/pgmj.2011.118398.

[2] Mokra D. 2021. "Acute Lung Injury – from Pathophysiology to Treatment." *Physiological Research*, January, S353-66. https://doi.org/10.33549/physiolres.934602.

[3] Ashbaugh DG, Bigelow DB, Petty TL and Levine BE. 1967. "Acute Respiratory Distress in Adults." *Lancet* (London, England), 2 (7511): 319-23. https://doi.org/10.1016/s0140-6736(67)90168-7.

[4] "Acute Respiratory Distress Syndrome." 2012. *JAMA,* 307 (23). https://doi.org/10.1001/jama.2012.5669.

[5] Confalonieri M, Salton F and Fabiano F. 2017. "Acute Respiratory Distress Syndrome." *European Respiratory Review,* 26 (144): 160116. https://doi.org/10.1183/16000617.0116-2016.

[6] Saguil A and Fargo MV. 2020. "Acute Respiratory Distress Syndrome: Diagnosis and Management." *American Family Physician*, 101 (12): 730-38. https://pubmed.ncbi.nlm.nih.gov/32538594/.

[7] Sweeney RM and McAuley DF. 2016. "Acute Respiratory Distress Syndrome." *The Lancet,* 388 (10058): 2416-30. https://doi.org/10.1016/s0140-6736(16)00578-x.

[8] Udobi KF, Childs E and Touijer K. 2003. "Acute Respiratory Distress Syndrome." *American Family Physician*, 67 (2): 315-22. https://pubmed.ncbi.nlm.nih.gov/12562153/.

[9] Parshall MB, Schwartzstein RM, Adams L, Banzett RB, Manning HL, Bourbeau J, Calverley PM, Gift AG, Harver A, Lareau SC, Mahler DA, Meek PM, O'Donnell DE. 2012. "An Official American Thoracic Society Statement: Update on the Mechanisms, Assessment, and Management of Dyspnea." *American Journal of Respiratory and Critical Care Medicine,* 185 (4): 435-52. https://doi.org/10.1164/rccm.201111-2042st.

[10] Burki, NK and Lee L-Y. 2010. "Mechanisms of Dyspnea." *Chest,* 138 (5): 1196-1201. https://doi.org/10.1378/chest.10-0534.

[11] Coccia CBI, Palkowski GH, Schweitzer B, Motsohi T and Ntusi N. 2015. "Dyspnea: Pathophysiology and a Clinical Approach." *South African Medical Journal,* 106 (1): 32. https://doi.org/10.7196/samj.2016.v106i1.10324.

[12] Petersson J and Glenny RW. 2014. "Gas Exchange and Ventilation–Perfusion Relationships in the Lung." *European Respiratory Journal*, 44 (4): 1023-41. https://doi.org/10.1183/09031936.00037014.

[13] Price LC, McAuley DF, Marino PS, Finney SJ, Griffiths MJ and Wort SJ. 2012. "Pathophysiology of Pulmonary Hypertension in Acute Lung Injury." *American Journal of Physiology - Lung Cellular and Molecular Physiology,* 302 (9): L803-15. https://doi.org/10.1152/ajplung.00355.2011.

[14] Spinelli E, Mauri T, Beitler JR, Pesenti A and Brodie D. 2020. "Respiratory Drive in the Acute Respiratory Distress Syndrome: Pathophysiology, Monitoring, and Therapeutic Interventions." *Intensive Care Medicine,* 46 (4): 606-18. https://doi.org/10.1007/s00134-020-05942-6.

Chapter 3

Lung Mechanics and Inflammatory Response

Laura Expósito Calamardo*, **MD**
Department of Cardiology,
Hospital Virgen de la Luz, Cuenca, Spain

Abstract

Ventilator induced lung injury (VILI) is acute lung damage caused or perpetuated by mechanical ventilation, both invasive and non-invasive. This lung damage is the product of different physical forces (pulmonary overdistention, pulmonary heterogeneity with areas of atelectasis, etc.) that will generate a series of mechanotransduction mechanisms and an inflammatory cascade responsible for the remodelling of the alveolocapillary membrane-edema and pulmonary fibrosis. Thus such as the translocation of inflammatory mediators and bacteria to the systemic circulation, generating multi-organ failure and patient death.

Keywords: ventilator induced lung injury (VILI), transpulmonary pressure, volutrauma, atelectrauma, biotrauma

Introduction

Mechanical ventilation is a fundamental tool in intensive care units for those patients with respiratory failure who require respiratory support. However, this ventilatory support is not without risks both at the pulmonary level and in the rest of the organs.

---

* Corresponding Author's Email: cascada.excal@gmail.com.

In: Ventilator Induced Lung Injury in Non-Invasive Ventilatory Support
Editor: Antonio M. Esquinas
ISBN: 979-8-88697-840-7

The first knowledge about lung damage induced by mechanical ventilation dates to 1744, when John Fothergill described that pulmonary resuscitation was better through mouth-to-mouth ventilation compared to machine bellows that generated the entry of air at high pressures and not controlled causing lung damage. Later, during the polio epidemic in 1952, the first studies began to publish on lung damage and the higher mortality rate in those patients who required mechanical respiratory support. Later, the concept of "respirator lung" defined to refer to the presence of extensive alveolar infiltrates and the formation of hyaline membranes in pathological samples of lungs under respiratory support [1]. However, the true importance of ventilator-induced lung injury established by studies published by the Acute Respiratory Distress Syndrome Network, which showed a relative reduction in the risk of death of 22% in those patients ventilated with a protective ventilation strategy pulmonary [2, 3].

Therefore, ventilation-induced lung injury (VILI) is the acute lung damage caused by mechanical ventilation, both invasive and non-invasive, and can appear in healthy lungs or perpetuate the situation of already existing lung damage. This phenomenon, as we will see below, is produced by different factors, both mechanical and biological, and which have implications at a systemic level.

Etiology

In a person undergoing treatment with mechanical ventilation, with an average respiratory rate of 15 rpm, the forces of lung stretching, and deformation occur an average of 21,600 times a day on 480 million alveoli. These repetitive changes in the tension and deformation of the alveoli during the respiratory cycles generate an inflammatory cascade that destroys the alveolar-capillary wall, thus causing lung damage and even the translocation of inflammatory mediators and bacteria to the systemic circulation, a phenomenon known as biotrauma [4, 5]. Among the main mechanical factors involved in this lung damage, barotrauma, volutrauma and atelectrauma will be considered.

Intrathoracic Pressures

During spontaneous breathing, the contraction of the inspiratory muscles and the mobilization of the chest wall generate a negative intrapleural pressure that allows lung expansion and the entry of air during inspiration. However, in a mechanically ventilated patient, it is necessary to generate a positive pressure that overcomes the resistance of the airway and the elastic properties of the lung. At the end of inspiration, in the zero-flow phase, the main force responsible for keeping the alveoli open is the transpulmonary pressure (alveolar pressure-pleural pressure). Lung volume and this transpulmonary pressure are closely related [6].

Barotrauma and Volutrauma

For years it has been thought that high intrathoracic pressures (barotrauma) were the main mechanism responsible for VILI. But from the study conducted by Dreyfuss et al., who used different ventilatory strategies in a group of rats, it was shown that pulmonary overdistention (volutrauma) is more important than barotrauma in generating damage to the pulmonary parenchyma [7].

When we subject an obese patient or a patient with a very rigid chest wall to mechanical ventilatory support, part of the positive pressure generated lost in trying to overcome the resistance offered by the chest wall and, therefore, the transpulmonary pressure generated will be lower, which leads to a lower entry of lung volume. However, for the same positive pressure on a patient with dyspnea and significant work of breathing, which generates an extremely negative intrapleural pressure due to respiratory effort, the transpulmonary pressure will be higher, leading to greater lung distention [6] (Figure 1).

It is these situations of high tidal volumes that are associated with the appearance of signs of barotrauma (pneumothorax, pneumomediastinum, subcutaneous emphysema) and VILI.

Atelectrauma

Ventilation on heterogeneous lungs, with areas of atelectasis (as occurs in acute respiratory distress syndrome) or during strategies with low total lung volumes, is also a cause of lung damage due to repetitive cycles of alveolar opening and collapse, which produces dysfunction of surfactant, loss of alveolar epithelium and formation of hyaline membranes. Phenomenon known as atelectrauma. The use of a positive pressure at the end of expiration, PEEP, has been shown to reduce lung damage induced by atelectrauma, by keeping the alveolar units open and thus reducing excessive alveolar deformation [6, 8].

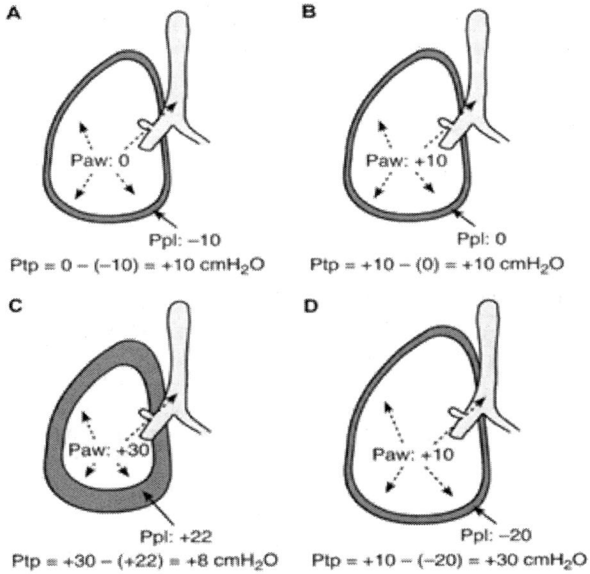

Abbreviations: Paw, airway pressure; Ppl, pleural pressure; Ptp, transpulmonary pressure.

Figure 1. Transpulmonary pressure (P airway-P pleural). Figures A-D represent the variation of Ptp in different clinical situations. A) During a spontaneous breath. B) Intubated patient without respiratory effort. C) Patient intubated but with a stiff chest wall. D) Intubated patient with asynchrony with the ventilator-respiratory effort. Jeremy R. Beitler et al. Ventilator-Induced Lung Injury. *Clin Chest Med.* 2016 December; 37(4): 633-646.

Biotrauma

Cytokines play a critical role in the inflammatory response and lung damage. They are produced by cells of the bronchial, bronchiolar, and alveolar epithelium, in addition to alveolar macrophages and neutrophils. Under normal conditions, there is a balance between proinflammatory cytokines (tumor necrosis factor-TNF-α, interleukin-IL I, IL-6, IL-8) and anti-inflammatory molecules (IL-10). Another fundamental element in the protection of the lung parenchyma is surfactant, whose levels decrease in the presence of the cytokines TNF-α and IL-1 [9].

Mechanical ventilation will produce an imbalance between these molecules, favoring the appearance of a proinflammatory cascade due to the previously described physical forces that generate changes by mechano-transduction (transcription of certain mechanosensitive genes). These mediators (TNF-α, IL-1β, IL-6, IL-8, and IL-10) and inflammatory cells (neutrophils, macrophages) trigger a loss of the alveolar-capillary membrane and therefore, the translocation of molecules, liposaccharides, and bacteria into the systemic circulation. This generates not only respiratory failure due to lung damage, but also extrapulmonary involvement of distant organs [8, 9] (Figure 2).

Other Mechanisms Involved

There are also other less described factors, but equally important, in the appearance of VILI:

- *Capillary stress failure.* During inspiration, pulmonary expansion decreases right ventricular filling, while during expiration it increases right ventricular filling and therefore the arrival of vascularization towards the pulmonary bed. These flow variations in the pulmonary vascular bed during respiratory cycles in patients with mechanical ventilation and especially with high volumes, will produce endothelial damage and microvascular leaks with leakage of water and proteins into the alveolar space (pulmonary edema) [10].
- *Lung deflation injury.* The sudden withdrawal of positive expiratory pressure (PEEP), as occurs during aspiration of respiratory secretions, disconnection of the tube or during patient transport, also favors the appearance of lung damage due to the sudden collapse of the alveolar units [10].
- *High-frequency oscillatory ventilation.* This is a ventilatory strategy that uses high respiratory rates and low tidal volumes, which theoretically would minimize lung injury. However, increasing respiratory rate could increase the deleterious effect on the lung due to increased cycling stress [11].

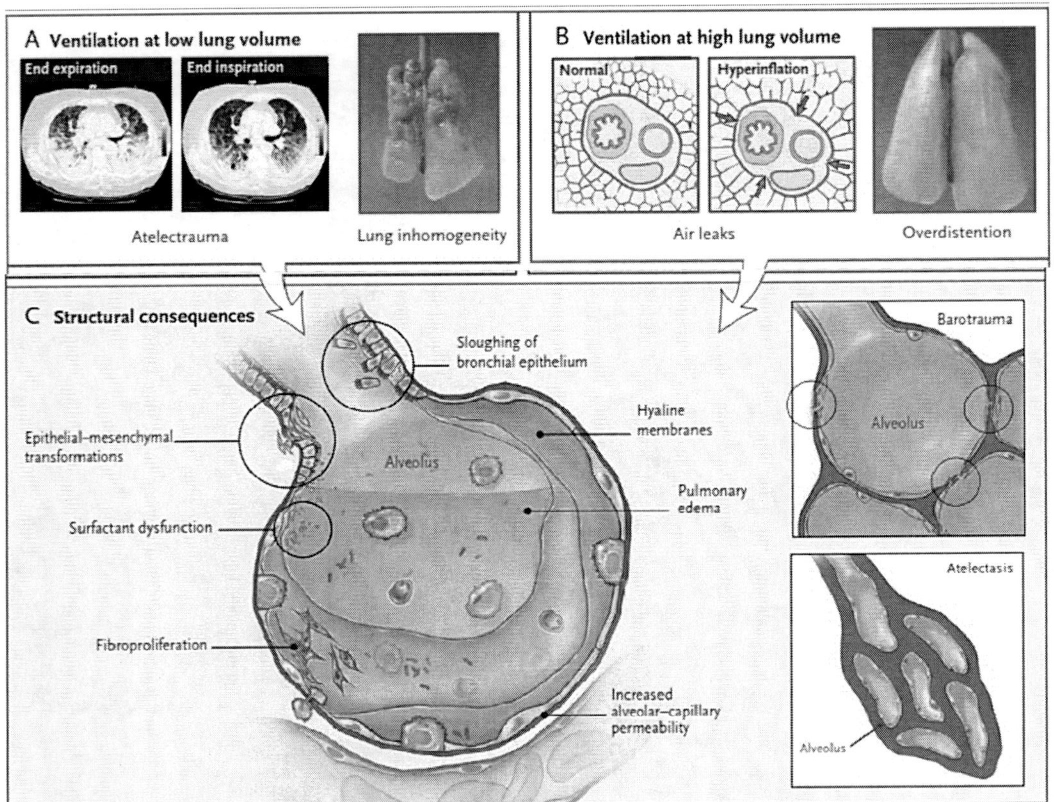

Figure 2. (Continued).

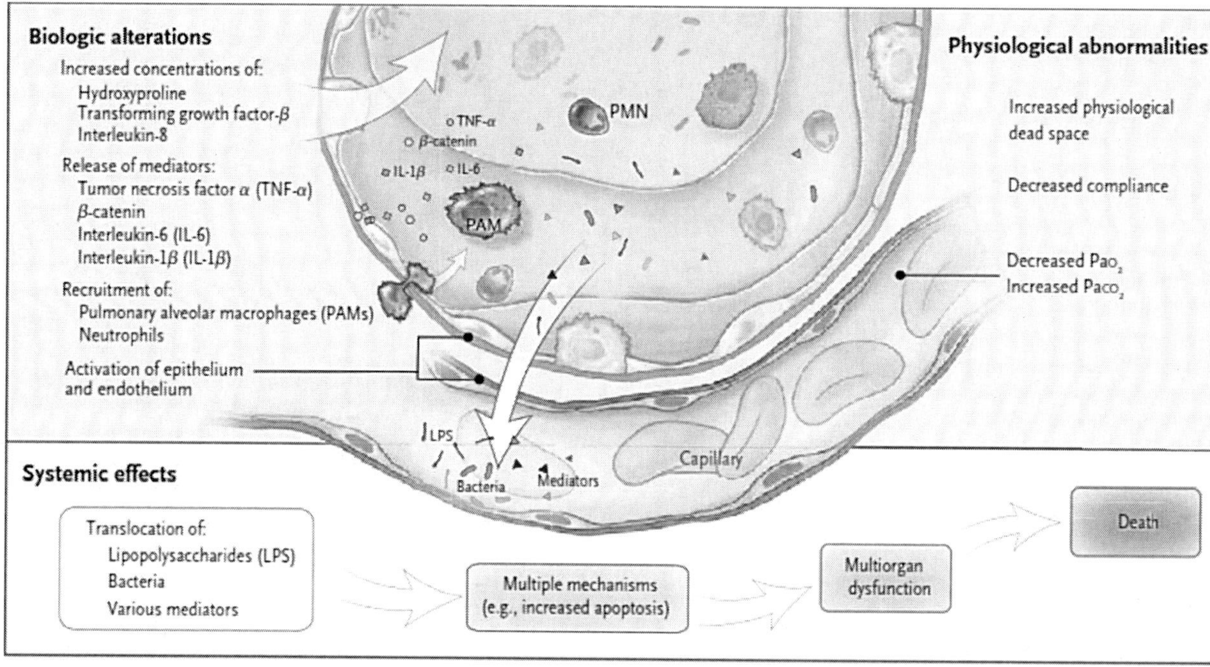

Figure 2. Lung injury caused by ventilation. Ventilation at low volumes (which will generate the appearance of atelectasis) (panel A) or with high tidal volumes (it will produce pulmonary overdistention) (panel B) will induce changes in the structure of the alveolar unit, such as the loss of the alveolar capillary membrane (panel C), due to the activation of an inflammatory cascade, which can spread to the extrapulmonary level and affect other organs. Arthur S. Slutsky et al. Ventilator-induced lung injury, *N Engl J Med* 2013; 369: 2126-36.

Lung Damage Induced by Non-Invasive Mechanical Ventilation

Patient-ventilator asynchrony has a negative impact on the appearance of lung damage. Those patients with acute pulmonary edema or exacerbated obstructive pulmonary disease, who find themselves with significant respiratory effort, will generate a very negative intrapleural pressure secondary to the effort of the inspiratory muscles, which will give rise to a high transpulmonary pressure and therefore, overdistention. A high expiratory volume >9.5 ml/Kg during non-invasive mechanical ventilation (resulting from respiratory effort) is an independent predictor of non-invasive ventilation failure and lung damage [10].

Conclusion

Mechanical ventilation, both invasive and non-invasive, can induce acute lung damage in healthy lungs or in already diseased lung tissue. Ventilatory strategies based on high tidal volumes (volutrauma) and the absence of PEEP (atelectrauma), favor the appearance of VILI.

The inflammatory cascade caused by ventilation not only generates lung damage but also extrapulmonary involvement (multi-organ failure syndrome). Patient-ventilator asynchrony generates higher transpulmonary pressure, and therefore pulmonary overdistention.

References

[1] Ajith Kumar AK, Fatima Anjum. *Ventilator-Induced Lung Injury (VILI)*. StatPearls [Pubmed]. Treasure Island (FL): StatPearls Publishing; 2022 Jan. 2021 Dec 15.

[2] The National Heart, Lung, and Blood Institute ARDS Clinical Trials Network. Higher versus Lower Positive End-Expiratory Pressures in Patients with the Acute Respiratory Distress Syndrome. *N Engl. J. Med.* 2004 Jul 22;351(4):327-36.

[3] The National Heart, Lung, and Blood Institute ARDS Clinical Trials Network. Ventilation with Lower Tidal Volumes as Compared with Traditional Tidal Volumes for Acute Lung Injury and the Acute Respiratory Distress Syndrome. *N. Engl. J. Med.* 2000; 342:1301-1308.

[4] Federico Gordo Vidal, C. Delgado Arnaiz and Eduaro Calvo Herranz. Mechanical ventilation induced lung injury. *Med. Intensiva*. 2007;31(1):18-26.

[5] Marini John, Gattinoni Luciano. Ventilatory management of acute respiratory distress syndrome: a consensus of two. *Crit. Care Med.* 2004; 32:250-5.

[6] Jeremy R. Beitler, Atul Malhotra, and Taylor Thompson. Ventilator-Induced Lung Injury. *Clin. Chest Med.* 2016 December; 37(4): 633-646.

[7] Didier Dreyfuss, Paul Soler, Guy Basset, and Georges Saumon. High inflation pressure pulmonary edema. Respective effects of high airway pressure, high tidal volume, and positive end-expiratory pressure. *Am. Rev. Respir. Dis.* 1988; 137(5): 1159-1164.

[8] Arthur S. Slutsky and Marco Ranieri. Ventilator-Induced Lung Injury. *N. Engl. J. Med.* 2013; 369: 2126-36.

[9] F. J. J. Halbertsma, M. Vaneker, G. J. Scheffer, J. G. van der Hoeven. Cytokines and biotrauma in ventilator-induced lung injury: a critical review of the literature. *Neth. J. Med.* 2005 Nov;63(10):382-92.

[10] Bhushan H Katira. Ventilator-Induced Lung Injury: Classic and Novel Cocepts. *Respir. Care* 2019;64(6):629-637.

[11] Hatchkiss JR, Blanch L, Murias G. Effects of decreased respiratory frequency on ventilator-induced lung injury. *Am. J. Respir. Crit. Care Med.* 2000;(161):463-8.

Chapter 4

Barotrauma, Volutrauma and Atelectrauma: Pathophysiology

Rosana Mara da Silva[1,*]
and Thales Cantelle Baggio[2]
[1] Respiratory Physiotherapy,
Hospital Municipal Health Department Jaraguá do Sul (SC), Brazil
[2] Cardiovascular Unit, Intensive Care Unit,
Hospital Jaraguá and Hospital São José, Jaraguá do Sul (SC), Brazil

Abstract

Several ventilation techniques have been studied and used to provide adequate respiratory support, but they can pose risk or damage to the lung parenchyma. Due to this possibility, it is necessary to understand the concept of some specific situations, such as barotrauma, volutrauma and atelectrauma, to identify potential risks and prevent their occurrence, especially in patients with severe respiratory syndromes. Thus, it is possible to recognize and avoid the ventilator-induced lung injury, so common in daily clinical practice.

Keywords: barotrauma, volutrauma, atelectrauma, pulmonar, ventilation

Introduction

The therapy of acute respiratory distress syndrome (ARDS) remains supportive, providing conditions for pulmonary healing with the lowest

---

[*] Corresponding Author's Email: rosanamara.fisio@gmail.com.

In: Ventilator Induced Lung Injury in Non-Invasive Ventilatory Support
Editor: Antonio M. Esquinas
ISBN: 979-8-88697-840-7

possible damage. Therefore, the choice of tidal volume and positive end-expiratory pressure (PEEP) levels primarily depends on the estimate of the risk associated with their application. The possible damages are collectively referred to as ventilator-induced lung injury (VILI) and their increase or decrease should represent the outcome variable when comparing different ventilatory modes [1].

While substantial evidence and consensus support the use of lower tidal volume to decrease VILI, the way of setting PEEP is more debated and controversial. Strategies of mechanical ventilation that place limits on airway pressure and tidal volume has been recommended for patients with the acute respiratory distress syndrome. Patients with the acute respiratory distress syndrome are particularly prone to overdistention, especially when conventional tidal volumes are used, because the number of lung units available for ventilation is markedly reduced as a result of fluid accumulation, consolidation, and atelectasis [2].

This chapter is focused on the concepts of barotrauma, volutrauma and atelectrauma, and the mechanical issues associated with these pathologies.

Definitions

Pulmonary barotrauma is a complication of mechanical ventilation and has correlations with increased morbidity and mortality. The natural mechanism of breathing in humans depends on negative intrathoracic pressures. However, patients on mechanical ventilation ventilate with positive pressures. Since positive pressure ventilation is not physiological, it may lead to complications such as barotrauma, which means the presence of extra alveolar air in locations where it is not present under normal circumstances. Barotrauma is most commonly due to alveolar rupture, which leads to an accumulation of air in extra alveolar locations. Excess alveolar air could then result in complications such as pneumothorax, pneumomediastinum, and subcutaneous emphysema [3].

Volutrauma refers to the local overdistention of normal alveoli. This concept has gained recognition over the last decades, and it is the reason for the use of lower tidal volumes of 6-8 mL/kg as a strategy of lung protection. When a mechanical ventilation breath is forced into the patient, the positive pressure tends to follow the path of least resistance to the normal or relatively normal alveoli, potentially causing overdistention. This overdistention sets off an inflammatory cascade that augments or perpetuates the initial lung injury, causing additional damage to previously unaffected alveoli. Another aspect of volutrauma associated with positive ventilation is the shear force associated with the opening and closing effects on collapsible alveoli. This has also been linked to worsening the local inflammatory cascade. PEEP prevents the alveoli from totally collapsing at the end of exhalation and may be beneficial in preventing this type of injury [4].

Studies performed with surfactant-depleted lungs on mechanical ventilation with various levels of PEEP provide support to the concept that the repeated opening and closing of terminal units causes additional injury, which is also a cause of VILI and described and called "atelectrauma." It seems likely that unstable lung units may be damaged by repeated opening and closing during tidal ventilation. PEEP may prevent diffuse alveolar damage during prolonged ventilation at high lung volume by stabilizing distal units. This may explain in part the preservation of alveolar epithelium integrity and the decrease in edema during high tidal volume mechanical ventilation in the presence of PEEP [5].

Pathophysiology

The inflammatory response to injury may include activation of macrophages that generate 'early response cytokines' like TNF-α and IL-1. These cytokines stimulate vascular endothelial cells to express vascular adhesion molecules, such as intercellular adhesion molecule-1 (ICAM-1), and E-selectin. Blood neutrophils adhere to endothelial cells and transmigrate into the interstitial and alveolar compartments. The entry of neutrophils into the alveolar compartment together with tissue-activated macro- phages sets the stage for injury of both lung cells and matrix glycoproteins (e.g., collagens, elastin). Injury is related to generation of oxidants by phagocytic cells and the release of proteases [5].

The acute respiratory distress syndrome constitutes acute hypoxemic respiratory failure after an inciting insult caused by a neutrophil-rich exudative pulmonary edema. Associated features include microvessel thrombi, increased permeability across both endothelial and alveolar epithelial layers, reduced fluid clearance, and protein-rich hyaline membrane formation. Subsequently, the diffuse alveolar damage of the acute phase will either gradually resolve, or progress as interstitial fibrosis, leading to pulmonary impairment. This syndrome remains defined clinically, without reliable biochemical or molecular diagnostics [6].

Conclusion

Positive pressure ventilation is commonly utilized in the management of patients with ARDS, which improves oxygenation and survival. The utilization of positive pressure predisposes an already diseased lung in ARDS to VILI [7].

It is clear that mechanical ventilation can damage the lungs when used with unappropriated configurations. Lesions at the alveolar–capillary interface, alterations in permeability, and edema have repeatedly been shown to occur in several studies due to adverse patterns of mechanical ventilation. In the last decades it was demonstrated that mechanical lung protection can be provided in patients with the acute respiratory distress syndrome, resulting in better pulmonary function and higher rates of weaning from the ventilator. Briefly, lung protection was based on a strategy of maintaining low inspiratory driving pressures, with the simultaneous circumvention of alveolar collapse using high PEEP to keep end-expiratory pressures above the lower inflection point on the static pressure-volume curve of the respiratory system. The nearly maximal alveolar recruitment and aeration accomplished with this strategy were intended to minimize shear stresses in the lung tissue during inspiration [8].

Another concerning factor is patient self-inflicted lung injury (P-SILI), which can induce lung injury as a consequence of intense inspiratory efforts. In patients with ARDS and acute hypoxemic respiratory failure, respiratory drive is increased. The intense inspiratory efforts generated therefore predispose to lung injury due to uncontrolled swings in trans-pulmonary pressure, which, in turn, abnormally increases lung stress and causes inflation of big tidal volumes. Alveolar rupture can lead to air leak, causing pulmonary interstitial emphysema, which can lead to pneumothorax, pneumomediastinum, and subcutaneous emphysema. This can be precipitated with an increase in intra-alveolar pressure due to any situation such as positive pressure ventilation, recruitment maneuver, coughing, or ventilator asynchrony [9].

The strong protective effect associated with a high PEEP value is consistent with recent experimental data, and the benefit seems to be more pronounced than the deleterious effect of high distending pressures. Recent evidence suggests that the minimization of ventilator-induced lung injury may have important systemic benefits, decreasing the release of proinflammatory mediators, the dissemination of infections, and possible complications related to air embolism. In addition to preventing progressive respiratory failure, the protective-ventilation approach may be associated with these mechanisms [10]. The protective-ventilation approach may thus not only improve pulmonary function and oxygenation but also reduce clinically apparent alveolar damage [11].

References

[1] Cipulli F., Vasques F., Duscio E., Romitti F., Quintel M., Gattinoni L. 2018. "Atelectrauma o volutrauma: the dilema." *Journal of Thoracic Disease* 10(3), 1258-1264. doi: https://doi.org/10.21037/jtd.2018.02.71.

[2] Stewart T. E., Meade M. O., Cook D. J., Granton J. T., Hodder R. V., Lapinsky S. E., Mazer C. D., McLean R. F., Rogovein T. S., Schouten B. D., Todd T. R., Slutsky A. S. 1998. "Evaluation of a ventilation strategy to prevent barotrauma in patients at high risk for acute respiratory distress syndrome. Pressure- and Volume-Limited Ventilation Strategy Group." *The New England Journal of Medicine*, 338(6), 355–361. https://doi.org/10.1056/NEJM199802053380603.

[3] Diaz R., Heller D. *Barotrauma and Mechanical Ventilation*. 2021. In: *StatPearls* [Internet]. Treasure Island (FL): StatPearls Publishing; 2021 Jan. https://www.ncbi.nlm.nih.gov/books/NBK545226/.

[4] Slutsky A. S., Ranieri V. M. 2013. "Ventilator-induced lung injury." *The New England Journal of Medicine*. 369(22), 2126-36. doi: https://doi.org/10.1056/NEJMra1208707. Erratum in: N Engl J Med. 2014 Apr 24;370(17):1668-9. PMID: 24283226.

[5] Attar M. A., Donn S. M. 2002. "Mechanisms of ventilator-induced lung injury in premature infants." *Seminars in Neonatology*. Oct; 7(5), 353-60. doi: https://doi.org/10.1053/siny.2002.0129. PMID: 12464497.

[6] Yehya N. 2019. "Lessons learned in acute respiratory distress syndrome from the animal laboratory." *Annals of Translational Medicine*. 7(19), 503. doi: https://doi.org/10.21037/atm.2019.09.33.

[7] Rajdev K., Spanel A. J., McMillan S., Lahan S., Boer B., Birge J., Thi M. 2021. "Pulmonary Barotrauma in COVID-19 Patients with ARDS on Invasive and Non-Invasive Positive Pressure Ventilation." *Journal of Intensive Care Medicine*. Sep, 36(9), 1013-1017. doi: https://doi.org/10.1177/08850666211019719. Epub 2021 May 20. PMID: 34013825.

[8] Amato M. B., Barbas C. S., Medeiros D. M., Magaldi R. B., Schettino G. P., Lorenzi-Filho G., Kairalla R. A., Deheinzelin D., Munoz C., Oliveira R., Takagaki T. Y., Carvalho C. R. 1998. "Effect of a protective-ventilation strategy on mortality in the acute respiratory distress syndrome." *The New England Journal of Medicine* Feb 5, 338(6), 347-54. doi: https://doi.org/10.1056/NEJM199802053380602. PMID: 9449727.

[9] Grieco D. L., Menga L. S., Eleuteri D., Antonelli M. 2019. "Patient self- inflicted lung injury: implications for acute hypoxemic respiratory failure and ARDS patients

on non-invasive support." *Minerva Anestesiologica*, 85(9), 1014–1023. https://doi.org/10.23736/S0375-9393.19.13418-9.

[10] Tremblay L., Valenza F., Ribeiro S. P., Li J., Slutsky A. S. 1997. "Injurious ventilatory strategies increase cytokines and c-fos m-RNA expression in an isolated rat lung model." *The Journal of Clinical Investigation* 99(5), 944–952. https://doi.org/10.1172/JCI119259.

[11] Gabrielli M., Valletta F., Franceschi F.; Gemelli Against COVID 2019. 2021. "Barotrauma during non-invasive ventilation for acute respiratory distress syndrome caused by COVID-19: a balance between risks and benefits." *British Journal of Hospital Medicine* (London) Jun 2, 82(6), 1-9. https://doi.org/10.12968/hmed.2021.0109.

Chapter 5

Non-Invasive Ventilation and Biotrauma: Pathophysiology

Aneesa S. Shahul[1,*], MD, DM, DNB, EDARM, MRC and B. L. Parvathi[2], MD

[1] Respiratory Medicine,
Ananthapuri Hospitals and Research Institute (AHRI), Kerala, India
[2] Pulmonology Department, ESI Hospital, Delhi, India

Abstract

Ventilator-induced lung injury (VILI) is the acute lung damage induced or intensified by mechanical ventilation. Release of inflammatory mediators from injured lung resulting in multi-organ injury is referred to as biotrauma. Mechanical overdistension, orthogonal stress and shear stress applied on the alveoli during non-invasive ventilation triggers the release of a plethora of inflammatory mediators. The major cells involved in this process are the polymorphonuclear cell (PMN) and the alveolar macrophage.

Biomarkers have the potential to identify patients at high-risk for VILI. Angiopoietin-2 is the most promising plasma biomarker for estimating endothelial injury. Von Willebrand factor (VWF), surfactant protein D and interleukin-6 are the other biomarkers under investigation for identifying biotrauma. Animal models have demonstrated the efficacy of therapies aimed at mitigating biotrauma. Role of prophylactic, inhaled IL-10 and intravenous delivery of anti-TNF antibodies is under trials in animal models. The use of mesenchymal stem cells (MSCs) which has the potential to impact on inflammation (and hence biotrauma) and augment tissue repair is a promising therapeutic strategy.

---

* Corresponding Author's Email: aneesambbs@gmail.com.

In: Ventilator Induced Lung Injury in Non-Invasive Ventilatory Support
Editor: Antonio M. Esquinas
ISBN: 979-8-88697-840-7

Keywords: ventilator-induced lung injury, mechano transduction, biotrauma, cytokine, MODS

Overview

Ventilator induced lung injury (VILI) is the acute lung damage induced or intensified by mechanical ventilation. [1]. Though widely discussed in the context of invasive mechanical ventilation, it can occur with non-invasively ventilated patients as well. To list down a few terms linked to this aspect:

1. *Barotrauma*: Inflation pressure related lung injury which can lead to pneumothorax and pneumomediastinum.
2. *Volutrauma*: Excessive stretch of alveoli due to high tidal volumes
3. *Biotrauma*: Release of inflammatory mediators from injured lung resulting in multi-organ injury.
4. *Myotrauma*: Deleterious structural changes occurring in the lung consequent to mechanical ventilation.
5. *Atelectotrauma*: Cyclical opening and closing of the alveoli leading to damage to non-atelectatic alveoli.

Pathophysiology

The biotrauma hypothesis has two parts:

1. Ventilation may cause release of mediators.
2. These mediators have biological actions [2].

Mechanical overdistension, orthogonal stress and shear stress applied on the alveoli during non-invasive ventilation triggers the release of a plethora of inflammatory mediators. This injury is propagated by the microenvironmental imbalance of pro and anti-inflammatory mediators. These mediators originating in the lung also gain access to the systemic circulation, terminating in multi-organ dysfunction and death [3, 4].

There are 4 principal mechanisms by which mediator release occurs after cyclic stretch:

1. Decompartmentalization which is the stress induced failure of the alveolar epithelial–endothelial barrier.
2. Stress necrosis of the plasma membrane.
3. Mechano transduction which means alterations in the cytoskeletal structure without ultrastructural damage.
4. Direct effects on vasculature.

Mechano transduction leads to functional changes in gene expression pattern, pro- and anti-inflammatory activity, alveolar epithelial barrier function and alveolar fluid clearance [5].

Cytopathology

The major cells involved in this process are the polymorphonuclear cell (PMN) and the alveolar macrophage. PMNs have been implicated as causative for both ALI and VILI. In rodent models, to a large extent, neutrophil migration into the alveoli appears to be dependent on stretch-induced macrophage inflammatory protein (MIP)-2 production from resident parenchymal cells. In rabbit models, cyclic overstretching of normal lungs with large Vt (20 ml/kg) is known to cause neutrophil influx and elevation in IL-8 levels in bronchoalveolar lavage (BAL) fluid [6]. Neutrophil depletion by vinblastine injection appears to attenuate IL-8 increase in the lung. P-selectin or intercellular adhesion molecule-1 (ICAM-1) are not expressed in animals depleted of neutrophils. These findings suggest that production of IL-8 by lung overstretch requires interaction between resident lung cells and migrated neutrophils. PMNs get activated after migration into alveolar space [7].

In a recent study, Belperio et al., demonstrated that the stress generated by mechanical forces enhances the PMN-induced changes in microvascular permeability in the lung. The ability of neutrophils to cause lung damage was mediated by increased expression of CXC chemokine receptor (CXCR)2 ligand in lung tissues (resident parenchymal cells) interacting with CXCR2 receptor on PMNs after mechanical injury [8].

Pressure cycled ventilation can cause human alveolar macrophages to release cytokines and proteases *in vitro*, and the effect is amplified by bacterial

LPS [9.10]. The ability of cyclic stretch to modulate specific immune function is not restricted to cells of myeloid origin [11]. In both alveolar epithelial cells and bronchial epithelial cells, cyclic stretch leads to increased expression of IL-8. Augmentation of this response is seen with co-stimulation with tumor necrosis factor (TNF)-α [12]. However, although the initial inciting event (mechanical ventilation) may be injurious, interaction between the innate immune system and mechanical injury may be required for the development of the full-blown lung injury phenotype of VILI.

Biomarkers in Biotrauma

Biomarkers have the potential to identify patients at high-risk for VILI or to identify patients most likely to benefit from a specific intervention, such as ultra-low tidal volume, lung protective ventilation. Angiopoietin-2 is the most promising plasma biomarker for estimating endothelial injury during ARDS, predicts the development of ALI in patients with sepsis identified in the emergency department; while the receptor for advanced glycation end products (RAGE) may provide the best assessment of the extent of lung epithelial injury [13, 14].

Von Willebrand factor (VWF) may be useful as a plasma marker of impending ARDS in patients with non-pulmonary sepsis [15]. VWF levels are elevated in the edema fluid and plasma of patients with ARDS and correlate with poor clinical outcomes [16]. While increases in other biochemical and inflammatory markers, including surfactant protein D and interleukin 6, correlate somewhat with lung injury and mortality, no simple biologic marker currently serves in the same diagnostic capacity, as do cardiac enzymes in evaluation of suspected acute myocardial infarction. [17].

Other mediators of inflammation like increased levels of TNF are detected in blood and BAL fluid in lung injury, but an association between TNF levels and the development of ARDS has not been found. Lipoxygenase products of arachidonic acid metabolism have been detected in pulmonary edema fluid, BAL fluid, plasma, and urine, and elastase has been detected in BAL fluid in the setting of lung injury [18]. Increased levels of IL-6 and thrombomodulin in those who had fewer ventilator-free days [19].

The Link between Biotrauma and Ventilogenomics

Evolving molecular approaches that examine the cellular response to stretch and injury may facilitate an even greater understanding of the contribution of biotrauma during critical illness, including identification of novel candidate mediators. A major research focus nowadays is the genetic factors that contribute to susceptibility and severity of VILI (Ventilogenomics). The application of microarray-based approaches to animals and *in vitro* models of VILI has been seen in recent literature [20]. Copland and colleagues ventilated mice with large tidal volumes and identified genes that were highly up-regulated, including the immediate-early response genes Nur77, Egr1, Btg2, and c-Jun [21].

Management of Biotrauma

Several studies have found plasma cytokine levels to be higher during large tidal volume ventilation and associated with the development of MODS, and persistent cytokine elevation in turn is associated with a poor outcome in patients with ARDS. In the future, a biomarker-driven approach could guide ventilator management. In the ARDS Network low tidal volume study, lower tidal volumes led to lower levels of plasma IL-6, IL-8, and TNFR1 over the first 1– 3 days [22]. Stuber and colleagues found increases in IL-6 within one hour of switching from a lung protective strategy to a less protective strategy; 5 hours later the patients were returned to the lung protective strategy, and IL-6 decreased one hour thereafter [23]. Plasma RAGE levels also changed within 1 hour of a recruitment maneuver in patients with diffuse ARDS [24]. Bedside point-of-care testing of circulating mediators could potentially be used to guide ventilator management.

Animal models have demonstrated the efficacy of therapies aimed at mitigating biotrauma. Prophylactic, inhaled IL-10 improved survival and reduced lung injury in a model of VILI induced by high airway pressures and these results may be due to inhibition of biotrauma [25]. Intravenous delivery of anti-TNF antibodies decreased lung edema due to high pressure ventilation, as well as reduced the ventilation-associated increase in gut permeability in a rat model [26]. Anti-biotrauma therapies could be administered prior to the inciting stimulus – mechanical ventilation. The use of mesenchymal stem cells (MSCs) which has the potential to impact on inflammation (and hence biotrauma) and augment tissue repair IA a promising therapeutic strategy [27,28]. A phase I study of MSCs in ARDS has been completed and a phase II study is underway [29, 30].

References

[1] AK A K, Anjum F. *Ventilator-Induced Lung Injury (VILI)* [Updated 2021 Dec 15]. In: StatPearls [Internet]. Treasure Island (FL): StatPearls Publishing.

[2] Santos C C, Zhang H, Liu M, Slutsky AS. Bench-to-bedside review: Biotrauma and modulation of the innate immune response. *Crit. Care*. 2005;9(3):280-286. doi:10.1186/cc3022.

[3] Curley G F, Laffey J G, Zhang H, Slutsky A S. Biotrauma and Ventilator-Induced Lung Injury: Clinical Implications. *Chest*. 2016;150(5):1109-1117. doi:10.1016/j.chest.2016.07.019.

[4] Spieth P M, Bluth T, Gama De Abreu M, Bacelis A, Goetz AE, Kiefmann R. Mechanotransduction in the lungs. *Minerva Anestesiol*. 2014;80(8):933-941.

[5] Tremblay L N, Slutsky A S. Ventilator-induced lung injury: from the bench to the bedside. *Intensive Care Med*. 2006;32(1):24-33. doi:10.1007/s00134-005-2817-8.

[6] Halberstam F J, Vaneker M, Scheffer G J, van der Hoeven J G. Cytokines and biotrauma in ventilator-induced lung injury: a critical review of the literature. *Neth. J. Med*. 2005;63(10):382-392.

[7] Jones H A, Clark R J, Rhodes C G, Schofield J B, Krausz T, Haslett C: *In vivo* measurement of neutrophil activity in experimental lung inflammation. *Am. J. Respir. Crit. Care Med.* 1994, 149:1635- 1639.

[8] Belperio J A, Keane M P, Burdick M D, Londhe V, Xue YY, Li K, Phillips R J, Strieter R M. Critical role for CXCR2 and CXCR2 ligands during the pathogenesis of ventilator-induced lung injury. *J. Clin. Invest.* 2002;110(11):1703-16.

[9] Dunn I, Pugin J. Mechanical ventilation of various human lung cells *in vitro*: identification of the macrophage as the main producer of inflammatory mediators. *Chest* 1999;116(1 Suppl):S95-7.

[10] Tremblay L, Valenza F, Ribeiro SP, Li J, Slutsky AS. Injurious ventilatory strategies increase cytokines and c-fos m-RNA expression in an isolated rat lung model. *J. Clin. Invest.* 1997;99(5):944-52.

[11] Mourgeon E, Isowa N, Keshavjee S, Zhang X, Slutsky AS, Liu M. Mechanical stretch stimulates macrophage inflammatory protein-2 secretion from fetal rat lung cells. *Am. J. Physiol. Lung Cell Mol. Physiol.* 2000;279(4):L699-706.

[12] Blahnik M J, Ramanathan R, Riley C R, Minoo P. Lipopolysaccharide-induced tumor necrosis factor-alpha and IL-10 production by lung macrophages from preterm and term neonates. *Pediatr. Res*. 2001;50(6):726-731. doi:10.1203/00006450-200112000-00016.

[13] Ashish Agrawal[1], Michael A Matthay, Kirsten N Kangelaris, John Stein, Jeffrey C Chu, Brandon M Imp, Alfredo Cortez, Jason Abbott, Kathleen D Liu, Carolyn S

Calfee . Plasma angiopoietin-2 predicts the onset of acute lung injury in critically ill patients. *Am. J. Respir. Crit. Care Med.* 2013;187(7):736-742.

[14] Calfee C S, Ware L B, Eisner M D, Parsons P E, Thompson BT, Wickersham N, Matthay MA; NHLBI ARDS Network. Plasma receptor for advanced glycation end products and clinical outcomes in acute lung injury. *Thorax.* 2008;63(12):1083-1089.

[15] Rubin D B[1], J P Wiener-Kronish, J F Murray, D R Green, J Turner, J M Luce, A B Montgomery, J D Marks, M A Matthay. Elevated von Willebrand factor antigen is an early plasma predictor of acute lung injury in nonpulmonary sepsis syndrome. *J. Clin. Invest.* 1990;86(2):474–480.

[16] Ware L B, Conner E R, Matthay M A. von Willebrand factor antigen is an independent marker of poor outcome in patients with early acute lung injury. *Crit. Care Med.* 2001;29:2325–2331.

[17] Lorraine B Ware[1], Tatsuki Koyama, D Dean Billheimer, William Wu, Gordon R Bernard, B Taylor Thompson, Roy G Brower, Theodore J Standiford, Thomas R Martin, Michael A Matthay, NHLBI ARDS Clinical Trials Network. Prognostic and pathogenetic value of combining clinical and biochemical indices in patients with acute lung injury. *Chest.* 2010;137:288–296.

[18] *Fishman's Pulmonary Diseases and Disorders*, Fifth Edition.2015;4593. Editor-in-Chief: Michael A. Grippi. Editors: Jack A. Elias, Jay A. Fishman, Robert M. Kotloff, Allan I. Pack, Robert M. Senior.

[19] Ashish Agrawal, Hanjing Zhuo, Sandra Brady, Joseph Levitt, Jay Steingrub, Mark D Siegel, Graciela Soto, Michael W Peterson, Mark S Chesnutt, Michael A Matthay, Kathleen D Liu. Pathogenetic and predictive value of biomarkers in patients with ALI and lower severity of illness: results from two clinical trials. *Am. J. Physiol. Lung Cell Mol. Physiol.* 2012;303:634–639.

[20] Curley G F, Laffey J G, Zhang H, Slutsky A S, Biotrauma and Ventilator Induced Lung Injury: Clinical implications, *Chest* (2016), doi: 10.1016/j.chest.2016. 07.019.

[21] Copland I B, Kavanagh B P, Engelberts D, McKerlie C, Belik J, Post M. Early changes in lung gene expression due to high tidal volume. *Am. J. Respir. Crit. Care Med.* 2003;168(9):1051-1059.

[22] Roy G Brower[1], Paul N Lanken, Neil MacIntyre, Michael A Matthay, Alan Morris, Marek Ancukiewicz, David Schoenfeld, B Taylor Thompson. Higher versus lower positive end-expiratory pressures in patients with the acute respiratory distress syndrome. *N. Engl. J. Med.* 2004;351(4):327-336.

[23] Stüber F, H Wrigge, S Schroeder, S Wetegrove, J Zinserling, A Hoeft, C Putensen. Kinetic and reversibility of mechanical ventilation-associated pulmonary and systemic inflammatory response in patients with acute lung injury. *Intensive Care Med.* 2002;28(7):834-841.

[24] Matthieu Jabaudon[1], Nacim Hamroun, Laurence Roszyk, Renaud Guérin, Jean-Etienne Bazin, Vincent Sapin, Bruno Pereira, Jean-Michel Constantin. Effects of a recruitment maneuver on plasma levels of soluble RAGE in patients with diffuse acute respiratory distress syndrome: a prospective randomized crossover study. *Intensive Care Med.* 2015;41(5):846-855.

[25] Hoegl S, Boost K A, Czerwonka H, Dolfen A, Scheiermann P, Muhl H, Zwissler B, Hofstetter C. Inhaled IL-10 reduces biotrauma and mortality in a model of ventilator-induced lung injury. *Respir. Med.* 2009;103(3):463-470.

[26] Benoit P Guery, David A Welsh, Nathalie B Viget, Laurent Robriquet, Patrice Fialdes, Carol M Mason, Gilles Beaucaire, Greg J Bagby, Remi Neviere. Ventilation-induced lung injury is associated with an increase in gut permeability. *Shock*. 2003;19(6):559- 563.

[27] Curley G F, Ansari B, Hayes M, Devaney J, Masterson C, Ryan A, Barry F, O'Brien T, Toole D O, Laffey J G. Effects of intratracheal mesenchymal stromal cell therapy during recovery and resolution after ventilatorinduced lung injury. *Anesthesiology*. 2013;118(4):924-932.

[28] Curley G F, Hayes M, Ansari B, Shaw G, Ryan A, Barry F, O'Brien T, O'Toole D, Laffey J G. Mesenchymal stem cells enhance recovery and repair following ventilator-induced lung injury in the rat. *Thorax*. 2012;67(6):496-501.

[29] Wilson J G, Liu K D, Zhuo H, Caballero L, McMillan M, Fang X, Cosgrove K, Vojnik R, Calfee CS, Lee J W. Mesenchymal stem (stromal) cells for treatment of ARDS: a phase 1 clinical trial. *Lancet Respir. Med.* 2015;3(1):24-32.

[30] Liu K D, Wilson J G, Zhuo H, Caballero L, McMillan M L, Fang X, Cosgrove K, Calfee C S, Lee J W, Kangelaris K N, Gotts J E, Rogers A J, Levitt J E, Wiener-Kronish J P, Delucchi K L, Leavitt A D, McKenna D H, Thompson B T, Matthay MA. Design and implementation of the START (STem cells for ARDS Treatment) trial, a phase 1/2 trial of human mesenchymal stem/stromal cells for the treatment of moderate-severe acute respiratory distress syndrome. *Ann. Intensive Care.* 2014;4:22.

Chapter 6

Positive End-Expiratory Pressure and Ventilator-Induced Lung Injury: Mechanisms and Clinical Recommendations

Greta Zunino[1,2], MD,
Denise Battaglini[1,*], MD,
Paolo Pelosi[1,2], MD
and Patricia R.M. Rocco[3]
[1] Anesthesia and Intensive Care, San Martino Policlinico Hospital, IRCCS for Oncology and Neurosciences, Genoa, Italy
[2] Department of Surgical Sciences and Integrated Diagnostics (DISC), University of Genoa, Genoa, Italy
[3] Laboratory of Pulmonary Investigation, Carlos Chagas Filho Institute of Biophysics, Federal University of Rio de Janeiro, Rio de Janeiro, Brazil

Abstract

Mechanical ventilation (MV) is a key supportive strategy to treat respiratory failure but may itself cause injury if improperly set. Injuries related to MV are known as ventilator-induced lung injury (VILI), which encompasses a spectrum of components: volutrauma, barotrauma, atelectrauma, and biotrauma. Mechanical power, defined as the total energy transferred to the lungs during MV, is a novel way to describe all the components of VILI.

Many randomized clinical trials have been conducted to study the best ventilator strategy to improve outcomes while avoiding the harmful effects of MV, especially in patients with the acute respiratory distress

* Corresponding Author's Email: battaglini.denise@gmail.com.

In: Ventilator Induced Lung Injury in Non-Invasive Ventilatory Support
Editor: Antonio M. Esquinas
ISBN: 979-8-88697-840-7

syndrome (ARDS). Among the components of MV that can contribute to VILI, positive end-expiratory pressure (PEEP) contributes to VILI primarily by causing overdistension of the alveoli. However, if patients are well selected and assigned to the correct ventilator strategy, PEEP could mitigate VILI and improve both ventilation and patient outcomes.

To maximize the beneficial effect of MV, patients with ARDS should be investigated and assigned to a specific ARDS phenotype; this is key to individualized treatment. In turn, individualization of treatment must necessarily involve the use of new methods – including novel bedside methods – to investigate the response of the patient's lung to MV, especially recruitment maneuvers and higher levels of PEEP.

Keywords: ventilator-induced lung injury, positive end-expiratory pressure, protective ventilation, the phenotype of ARDS, mechanical power

Introduction

Mechanical ventilation (MV) is widely used as a supportive strategy in patients admitted to the intensive care unit (ICU) for various reasons, from chronic respiratory failure to acute respiratory failure (ARF), especially when the acute respiratory distress syndrome (ARDS) occurs [1]. Since the earliest days of MV, ventilator settings have been investigated to assess the best parameters to limit respiratory failure, while more recently researchers are focusing on the extent to which MV can have a beneficial impact on patient outcomes. MV could itself cause lung damage, which is then known as ventilator-induced lung injury (VILI); hence, a current matter of debate is how MV causes VILI and how VILI can be prevented.

Among patients who need MV, those that develop ARDS are most at risk of developing VILI because of the loss of cell-membrane integrity, associated edema, and presence of atelectatic regions, thus leading to a reduction of lung compliance. The forces applied by MV in atelectatic areas are responsible for the continuous opening and closing of alveoli, a potentially harmful mechanism [1]. Another mechanism of VILI includes the high inspiratory forces produced by the ventilator, which can stress the lung parenchyma with overdistension [2].

The application of positive end-expiratory pressure (PEEP) in patients with ARDS has knowns advantages, such as improved arterial oxygenation, transpulmonary shunt, and recruitment of collapsed alveoli [1]. Besides, PEEP can also play a crucial role in preventing and causing VILI. When appropriately set, PEEP avoids the opening and collapse of alveoli during the breathing cycle, maintaining recruitment (or end-expiratory lung volume – EELV). On the other hand, when PEEP itself generates an overdistension of the alveoli, it contributes to the augmentation of the stress forces applied to the lungs [2]. The purpose of this chapter is to elucidate the pathophysiology of PEEP-related VILI and the management of PEEP during MV to prevent VILI.

Pathophysiological Role of PEEP in VILI Atelectrauma

In ARDS, lungs are mechanically very heterogeneous. Injury to the alveolar-capillary interface leads to the accumulation of edema in both alveolar and interstitial spaces, with the collapse of the most dependent areas of the lungs, where atelectasis and consolidations prevail. The "sponge model" describes how the lungs are afflicted by ARDS: imagine the lungs as a sponge soaked in water; the normal (non-injured) lung parenchyma in the non-dependent areas has the best aeration (i.e., the "baby lung"), dependent areas are characterized by atelectasis (close areas, potentially openable); and consolidated areas are spread diffusely across the lungs, but more consistently in the dependent area [1]. As a result of all those changes, a reduced number of alveoli are available for ventilation, lung compliance decreases, and gas exchange worsens, with different grades of decrease in the arterial oxygen tension/inspiratory oxygen fraction ratio (PaO_2/FiO_2) [1]. MV can cause VILI when exaggerated forces are applied to the lung parenchyma, and ARDS represents an ideal lung model to predispose to such injury.

Lungs are more exposed to VILI when they are damaged or non-equally ventilated. High airway pressure and tidal volume (V_T) could be responsible for macroscopic injuries causing pneumothorax and pneumomediastinum [2]. High airway pressure, particularly transpulmonary pressure (P_L), is commonly identified as the *stress* component, while V_T is the *strain* component, meaning the volume variation (ΔV) above the resting lung volume or functional residual capacity (FRC). Both factors are components of the following formula: *strain* = *k* * *stress*, where *k* is the specific elastance (in males: 12-13 cmH_2O) [1].

Excessive stress on the lungs, such as volume (volutrauma) or pressure (barotrauma), leads to exaggerated and non-physiological strain, with consequent VILI. When the V_T is applied over an already distended lung (the lung volume at the total lung capacity), overdistension occurs with damage to the extracellular matrix and vessels and activation of inflammatory pathways [1]. Additionally, because of the inhomogeneity of the lungs in ARDS, the stress applied in the regions where open alveoli are close to the ones collapsed or filled with edema (close areas with different elasticity) seems to generate extra strain across the alveoli, with inflammation and damage of the residual healthy lung tissue (the "baby lung").

Of note, lung inhomogeneity becomes worse as ARDS worsens, which makes the lungs more vulnerable to VILI [2]; this mechanism is part of the so-called atelectrauma [1], and can also manifest when the collapsed alveoli cyclically open and close during the breathing cycle in response to stress, with impairment in surfactant function [1]. When MV triggers those mechanisms, inflammatory mediators are released by the damaged lungs, with biotrauma and systemic multiorgan involvement [2].

The concepts of stress and strain lead to the more recent idea of energy load on the lung parenchyma, defined as *mechanical power*, a parameter conceived with the purpose of providing a single number that can measure VILI comprehensively. The amount of energy applied to the respiratory system is derived from the equation of motion and is composed of three elements: (1) elastic energy: due to elastic recoil of the lung, linked to V_T and driving pressure; (2) resistance energy: due to the passage of flow in the airways; (3) elastic static energy: the lungs have their volume and pressure as a consequence of the PEEP at the beginning of the inspiration.

PEEP is not cycling applied in every breath (as, for example, V_T), but it is the pressure present in the lungs at the beginning of inspiration, which contributes to the energy sustained by the respiratory system. As all components of mechanical power, PEEP can contribute to VILI [1]. Negative effects of PEEP on the static strain applied on the lungs include that PEEP can recruit the collapsed alveoli or cause overdistension of those that are already open (or a mixture of both effects); when the latter effect prevails, PEEP causes an increase of EELV and static strain, and, so, of the total energy imparted to the respiratory system, with consequent tissue damage and inflammation [2].

Moreover, PEEP influences the cardiac output; when set above certain levels it can reduce cardiac output by raising the right arterial pressure with a reduced venous return and by increasing pulmonary vascular resistance, because it increases the P_L. PEEP can also enlarge the dead space when it is responsible for the augmentation of intra-alveolar pressure that overcomes pulmonary capillary pressure, with resulting hypoperfusion [2]. PEEP has also beneficial effects; it recruits collapsed lung units, making them available for ventilation and even perfusion (ventilation makes those areas no longer hypoxic; hypoxic vasoconstriction thus resolves, with consequent improvement of perfusion), improving intrapulmonary shunt, gas exchange, and arterial oxygenation [1], and avoiding cyclic opening and closing of the alveoli during ventilation, counteracting atelectrauma [2]. Recruiting lung units for ventilation reduces the dynamic strain, as the V_T can then be applied to a more open (i.e., compliant) lung, with mitigation of volutrauma [1].

Different studies have also reported distinct effects of PEEP on pulmonary edema; some proved that the increasing level of PEEP contributes to lung edema while others reported an indirect protective effect of PEEP on edema, as it reduces cardiac output and pulmonary blood volume [1]. The amount of negative versus positive effects of PEEP is difficult to establish a priori, because the number of recruitable lung units changes from patient to patient. The application of PEEP could lead to positive and negative effects and outcomes, and research continues to find the optimal PEEP. In the following sections, we will summarize the "state of the art" regarding PEEP settings based on the available evidence and future directions.

Clinical Considerations: Clinical Trials on PEEP in ARDS

Over the years, several clinical trials have been conducted to investigate the potential negative effect of mechanical ventilation on outcomes in patients with ARDS. In the ALVEOLI randomized clinical trial (RCT) [3], patients with acute lung injury (ALI) and ARDS were separated into two groups: higher versus lower PEEP approach. In the first group, PEEP was chosen based on the investigator's and clinician's analysis of the balance of beneficial and adverse effects; in the latter, PEEP was set starting from the findings of a previous study of the same group in which high PEEP levels and low V_T were associated to better survival. In the high-PEEP group, a level of at least 12 cmH_2O PEEP was maintained for 12 hours after randomization. The other MV parameters were the same in both groups: V_T of 6 ml/kg of predicted body weight (PBW) and inspiratory plateau pressure (P_{PLAT}) of 30 cmH_2O maximum. The results showed no significant differences in survival and days of unassisted breathing in the first 28 days.

The LOVS RCT [4] enrolled patients with ALI and ARDS and separated them into an open-lung ventilator strategy and control ventilation strategy. In the open-lung group, the expected ventilator settings were pressure control mode, V_T 6 ml/kg PBW, $P_{PLAT} < 40$ cmH_2O, a recruitment maneuver (RM), and a PEEP level adjusted following FiO_2, with modification in the PEEP level to set the higher level in this group. Patients of the control ventilation strategy were ventilated in volume-assist control mode, with a $P_{PLAT} < 30$ cmH_2O, and no possibility of RM; all other parameters were as in the open-lung group. The study showed no significant differences in mortality or incidence of barotrauma between the groups. The open-lung approach reduced the need for rescue therapies and was associated with fewer deaths due to refractory hypoxemia.

Patients with ALI were studied in the ExpPress RCT [5], the aim of which was to compare the impact of two different PEEP strategies on mortality. Both strategies established a V_T of 6 ml/kg PBW; patients selected for the minimal distension strategy received a moderate PEEP (5-9 cmH_2O), trying to maintain the lowest PEEP level possible to preserve oxygenation, while in the increased recruitment strategy, the PEEP was set as high as possible with the maximum limit of P_{PLAT} 28-30 cmH_2O. Mortality did not differ in the two groups, but the advantages of a recruitment overdistension-limiting strategy were a reduction in MV days, reduced organ failure, and improvement in oxygenation and lung compliance. Furthermore, the recruitment approach was not associated with a higher risk of barotrauma. A systematic review reanalyzed the independent data for the above-mentioned clinical trial and found that higher levels of PEEP were associated with better survival only in the subgroup of patients with moderate and severe ARDS [6].

The OLA RCT compared the data of patients with ARDS managed with the open-lung approach or the ARDS network protocol [7]. PEEP level was set using the decremental PEEP trial after an RM in the first group while, in the latter, PEEP was set using the FiO_2-PEEP table without RMs. The open-lung approach was not superior in reducing mortality, barotrauma, or ventilator-free days among patients with ARDS, but it improved oxygenation and driving pressure.

In the ART RCT [8], patients with moderate to severe ARDS in the intervention arm underwent an RM with incremental PEEP levels followed by a PEEP decrease according to the best respiratory system static compliance and another RM, while the control arm was managed with a low PEEP approach. The intervention group showed significantly higher 28-day mortality, with a hazard ratio of 1.22 (p-value 0.03) compared to the control group. The 7-day mortality was higher in the intervention group, with a greater number of deaths with barotrauma and a higher incidence of pneumothorax needing drainage. All-cause mortality was also higher in the experimental group than in the control group [8].

Patients with moderate to severe ARDS were enrolled in the PHARPAP trial [9] to study maximal lung recruitment that could improve the number of ventilator-free days. In the experimental group, patients underwent a maximal RM with PEEP titration, pressure-control ventilation with V_T 4-6 ml/kg PBW and P_{PLAT} 28 cmH_2O maximum; in the control group (control protective), ventilation was set in a volume-control mode with low V_T (4-6 ml/kg PBW), P_{PLAT} lower than 30 cmH_2O, and low PEEP. The study showed no improvement in ventilator-free days at 28 days nor mortality, but an increased incidence of cardiovascular adverse events; however, in the experimental group, the use of rescue therapies for hypoxemia was lower.

The current guidelines for mechanical ventilation in adult patients with ARDS [10] summarize and balance all the available data from clinical trials and other studies; higher versus lower PEEP does not improve survival and yields no significant differences in barotrauma, ventilator-free days, or organ failure, but oxygenation (PaO_2/FiO_2) is significantly higher in patients ventilated with high PEEP levels. The recommendations also consider the results of the aforementioned meta-analysis and ultimately suggest that adult patients with moderate to severe ARDS should be ventilated with high PEEP levels. Moreover, due to the influence of PEEP on inspiratory P_{PLAT}, the PEEP level should be titrated individually in every patient, especially when P_{PLAT} is greater than 30 cmH_2O – keeping the risk-benefit balance in mind [10].

Future Directions

The new era of personalizing MV in patients with ARDS will necessarily require identification of the distinct patterns, or phenotypes, of this condition. Always bearing in mind the Berlin definition of ARDS and its corresponding criteria [10], as well as the different grades of injury that can afflict the alveolar-capillary interface [1, 11] the subsequent step will be identification of radiological patterns of ARDS and predictable lung recruitability [11]. A recent series of articles in *The Lancet,* [11] proposed the classification of ARDS patients into different phenotypes: etiological (pulmonary or extrapulmonary); biological (hypo inflammatory or hyperinflammatory); physiological (based on the response to recruitment, assessed by shunt fraction and dead space using quantitative computed tomography [CT]); and radiological [11]. We will focus on the latter classification.

ARDS patients can be separated into two categories based on the morphological aspect of the lungs on CT scan performed at a PEEP level of 5

cmH_2O: (1) lungs with diffuse and heterogenous loss of aeration, the "diffuse/patchy pattern"; or (2) lungs with prevalent consolidation in the dorsal and lower sections, the "focal pattern" [11]. Patients with the "focal pattern" on CT show minimal loss of lung volume, contained augmentation of lung weight, and poor alveolar recruitment with increased hyperinflation after the application of PEEP [12] but a good gas-exchange response to prone positioning [11]. Patients with the "diffuse/patchy" (also known as "non-focal") pattern, in turn, showed a greater loss of lung volume, increased lung weight, and response to PEEP with higher lung recruitment [11, 12]. Indeed, driving pressures are higher in the diffuse pattern.

Correct individuation of lung morphology and allocation of patients to the best treatment strategy could benefit from a rapid, widely available, radiation-free bedside tool: lung ultrasound (LUS), which also avoids the risk of transporting unstable patients to the CT scanner. Recent data suggest that LUS is reliable in the identification of aerated regions and morphology patterns compared to chest CT [12]; with that knowledge, bedside ventilation management could use LUS findings to adapt MV to the rapidly progressing clinical condition of patients with ARDS.

A recent *post hoc* analysis [13] tested the accuracy of LUS in assessing lung morphology in patients with ARDS, compared with chest CT as the standard of care. Three different methods were analyzed: in the Lombardy method, LUS was performed just before chest CT, with the same ventilator settings for both scans (PEEP level = 5 cmH_2O), while in the Amsterdam method, LUS was performed in the ICU before transfer to the CT scanner; ventilator settings were maintained based on clinical titration. In both methods, LUS was acquired using a 12-region protocol with the patient in a semi-recumbent position; a score was assigned to each region according to a different pattern of visualized artifacts, and the sum score of all regions was calculated.

The third method, the previously validated Piedmont method, defined lungs with a LUS score ≤ 2 as a "non-focal" pattern and all others as focal pattern. Results showed moderate to good accuracy of the tested methods in predicting lung morphology: the Piedmont method had a sensitivity of 91% and a specificity of 75%, the Amsterdam method had a sensitivity of 77% and a specificity of 100%, and the Lombardy method had a sensitivity of 100% and a specificity of 61%, while the ROC curve of the anterior LUS score established the cutoff for identification of the non-focal phenotype as ≤ 2 regions in both the Lombardy and Amsterdam methods [13]. In the Amsterdam cohort, the lateral LUS score was higher in patients with a non-focal morphology pattern than in those with focal morphology, but this result was not reproducible in the Lombardy cohort, and the posterior LUS score did not differ between the different morphology patterns [13]. Anterior LUS scores highly influence the classification of lung morphology, and a low score in those regions (that classifies the morphology as "non-focal") could suggest the use of low PEEP and prone positioning, avoiding RM [13].

Radiological Phenotypes

Within the context of radiological phenotypes of ARDS, it is becoming even more important to identify patients who can benefit from PEEP and RM to limit harm and improve outcomes. Improvement of oxygenation in response to the application of higher PEEP levels could be a parameter to identify patients who can benefit from PEEP; secondary analysis of a recent study [14] showed how, in patients randomized to receive high PEEP, increasing PaO_2/FiO_2 ratio was associated with reduced mortality, consistent with the findings of the ExpPress RCT [5]. Those findings are possibly due to the recruitment effect of PEEP [2]; however, setting PEEP levels based on oxygenation still needs more evidence to prove its accuracy. Recent Bayesian network meta-analysis [15] evaluated the effect of PEEP and RM in moderate and severe ADRS. Interestingly, higher PEEP without RM was more beneficial than a lower PEEP strategy in terms of mortality, while high PEEP plus RM is more dangerous than a high PEEP strategy without RM, increasing mortality.

Assessing Individualized Recruitability

Before starting MV could guide the appropriate choice of PEEP, improving outcomes and avoiding harm in patients with ARDS, but this is not easy to achieve in practice. Different methods have been tested to identify lung recruitment; previously, we anticipated that improvement in oxygenation in response to PEEP is partly due to the recruitment effect, but other factors contribute, such as the positive effect of PEEP on cardiac output (it reduces the transmural left ventricular pressure, thus reducing left ventricular afterload) [2]. The combination of physiologic variables (PaO_2/FiO_2 ratio and respiratory system compliance, C_{rs}, at 5 and 10 cmH_2O PEEP levels) can be used to predict higher lung recruitment [16]. CT scan can identify different density shapes in the lungs, interpreted as diverse levels of tissue aeration; comparing the aspect of the lungs at different PEEP levels could reveal the amount of lung newly inflated as an effect of recruitment [2].

As noted above, identification of physiological phenotypes is based on the analysis of data from quantitative CT plus evaluation of shunt fraction and dead space. The recruitable phenotype has a lower PaO_2/FiO_2 ratio and C_{rs}, higher dead space and suboptimal inflated lung, and higher mortality; an increase of PEEP from 5 cmH_2O to 15 cmH_2O in those patients significantly improves lung aeration and PaO_2/FiO_2 ratio, dead space, and C_{rs} [11]. Conversely, the application of high PEEP in patients with poor recruitability causes an augmentation of static stress and strain, with undesired cardiovascular effects, VILI, and biotrauma [16].

Helium and nitrogen washout techniques at different PEEP levels can be used to assess the EELV as a measure of recruitment; these measurements could contribute to titrating the safest PEEP, as demonstrated by the ongoing multicenter IPERPEEP trial [17], an RCT which aims to choose the correct PEEP level based on the individualized measurement of lung recruitability in ARDS patients. The EELV and inspiratory capacity (IC) could be used to target V_T more accurately than setting V_T based on PBW (because of the lung heterogeneity in ARDS), aiming for protective MV, but this method is influenced by the level of PEEP [12]. When a high PEEP is set, EELV could change the C_{rs}, leading to inappropriate V_T targeting, while IC may not be influenced. At lower PEEP levels, IC is more reliable than EELV and V_T could be chosen based on EELV [12]. Increasing PEEP in a non-recruitable lung produces overdistension, increasing EELV, while in a recruitable the effect on the EELV is the same but with a more feasible effect: aeration of the already aerated alveoli plus reopening of the collapsed lung units; only in the first case is the effect on lung structure dangerous.

Targeting VT on the basis of IC considers the recruitability of the lung in theory, but in practice, IC and EELV are strictly correlated in ARDS [12]. Additionally, the ART trial [8] proved that, when PEEP is set so as to maximize C_{rs}, limiting driving pressure, the patient's survival decreases in comparison to a low PEEP approach. Those findings are linked to the fact that C_{rs} and driving pressure are measurements of the global behavior of the lung, while in ARDS the heterogeneity and the interaction between different sections of the lung are essential [9, 18]. Even though the idea of personalizing PEEP based on the amount of individual recruitment is physiologically sound, evidence suggests that PEEP-induced changes in C_{rs} and driving pressure are inaccurate measures of the amount of recruitment.

Recent findings prove that lung recruitment at CT scan was not systematically correlated to an increased C_{rs}, nor that the unchanged C_{rs} predict the absence of lung recruitment; the same correlation is proved for driving pressure [18]. A novel approach to personalizing MV is oriented to the use of P_L, given its importance in lung injury. Esophageal manometry (EM) can estimate the pleural pressures, and thus, measure P_L; high pleural pressure may indicate high P_L at the end of the expiration with the risk of lung collapse [19]. With EM, monitoring P_L with the goal of a positive value, PEEP could be set correctly to avoid decruitment, cycling opening, closing of the alveoli during ventilation, and decreasing atelectasis; the overall effect of this titration strategy is an optimized lung mechanic and oxygenation [19]. However, this method is not completely free of impurities: positional artifacts, distortion, esophageal contraction, and heterogeneity in pleural pressure in the respiratory system (a single point measurement may be not representative).

Nevertheless, EM has shown its reliability in estimating the P_L [19]. Lung recruitment could be assessed by electrical impedance tomography (EIT), a bedside method that scans ventilation and perfusion in real time by measuring the current conductivity throughout the thorax and respiratory system, detecting recruitment, overdistension, and changes in ventilated lung regions during the breathing cycle [12]. The increased volume of air in the lungs causes a reduction in current conductivity, with an increase in impedance; the study of impedance detects different aerated areas (from collapsed to overdistended) and the change of impedance could estimate the distribution of V_T throughout the heterogeneity of the lungs [16].

EIT confrontation of different lung impedances after different applications of PEEP could help predict lung recruitment [2]: the impedance change reflects the aeration gain or loss (as recruitment or overdistension) and can be used to direct RM, as well as to identify recruitable and non-recruitable patients [16]. Rezoagli and Bellani proposed a two-step, EIT-based PEEP titration strategy: after a diagnostic RM aimed to assess the potential lung recruitability, the PEEP level is increased stepwise in small increments until the level that permits a stable value of EELV, assessed by the impedance signal at the end of expiration [16]. The results of this approach were an improvement in oxygenation and a reduction of driving pressure, as well as providing data on alveolar overdistension or collapse of lung regions [16]. Figure 1 summarizes the methods available to assess PEEP at bedside.

The LIVE RCT [20] showed the importance of the correct allocation of patients into groups: only patients who were correctly classified benefited from the personalized MV approach, with a 10% decrease in mortality, while misclassification was associated with an increase in mortality.

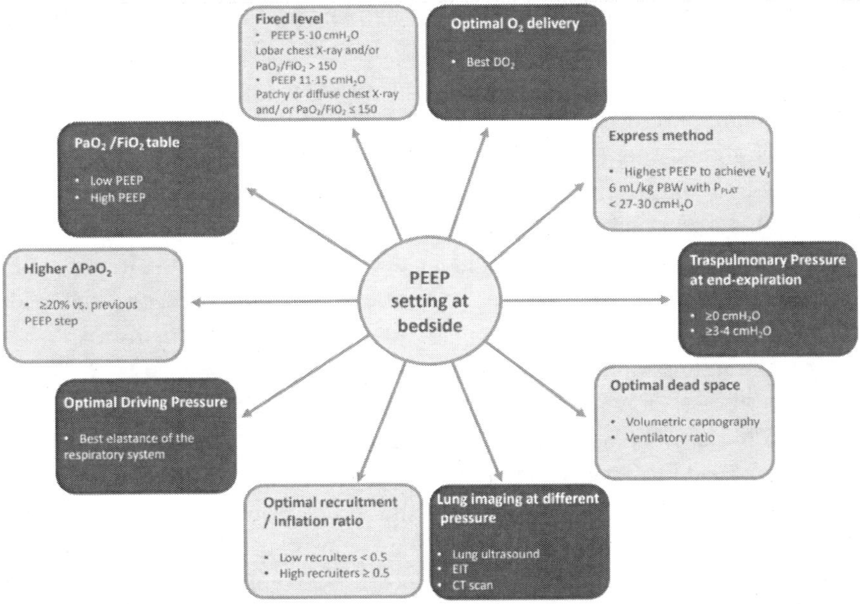

Figure 1. Summary of the bedside methods to set PEEP. Positive end-expiratory pressure (PEEP), ratio of arterial oxygen partial pressure to fraction of inspired oxygen (PaO_2/FIO_2), Oxygen delivery (DO_2), electrical impedance tomography (EIT), chest computed tomography (CT) scan, predicted body weight (PBW), tidal volume (V_T), plateau pressure *(P_{PLAT})*.

Conclusion

What strongly emerges from the literature and the available knowledge is that MV is a lifesaving therapy but is not free from causing harmful effects, known as VILI; achieving the first while avoiding the latter is a continuous challenge. Among the components of MV, we analyzed the role of PEEP, which can have both beneficial and undesired effects; for the time being, there is no one method that can assess the best PEEP or predict its effects but is clear that this component should be titrated individually. Heterogeneity in patient and illness characteristics, especially in the case of ARDS, surely contributes to the complexity of predicting the effects of MV. Future studies and clinical trials would do well to investigate subgroups of ARDS patients in the pursuit of personalized ventilator strategies [1, 15].

References

[1] Pelosi P., Rocco P. R. M., and Gama de Abreu M., "Close down the lungs and keep them resting to minimize ventilator-induced lung injury," *Crit. Care*, vol. 22, p. 72, Mar. 2018, doi: 10.1186/s13054-018-1991-3.

[2] Sahetya S. K., Goligher E. C., and Brower R. G., "Fifty Years of Research in ARDS. Setting Positive End-Expiratory Pressure in Acute Respiratory Distress Syndrome," *Am. J. Respir. Crit. Care Med.*, vol. 195, no. 11, pp. 1429–1438, Jun. 2017, doi: 10.1164/rccm.201610-2035CI.

[3] Brower R.G., Lanken P.N., MacIntyre N., Matthay M.A., Morris A., Ancukiewicz M., Schoenfeld D., Thompson B.T.; National Heart, Lung, and Blood Institute ARDS Clinical Trials Network. "Higher versus Lower Positive End-Expiratory Pressures in Patients with the Acute Respiratory Distress Syndrome," *N. Engl. J. Med.*, vol. 351, no. 4, pp. 327–336, Jul. 2004, doi: 10.1056/NEJMoa032193.

[4] Meade M. O., Cook D. J., Guyatt G. H., Slutsky A. S., Arabi Y. M., Cooper D. J., Davies A. R., Hand L. E., Zhou Q., Thabane L., Austin P., Lapinsky S., Baxter A., Russell J., Skrobik Y., Ronco J. J., and Stewart T. E., for the Lung Open Ventilation Study Investigators, "Ventilation Strategy Using Low Tidal Volumes, Recruitment Maneuvers, and High Positive End-Expiratory Pressure for Acute Lung Injury and Acute Respiratory Distress Syndrome: A Randomized Controlled Trial," *JAMA*, vol. 299, no. 6, pp. 637–645, Feb. 2008, doi: 10.1001/jama.299.6.637.

[5] Mercat A., Richard J.-C. M., Vielle B., Jaber S., Osman D., Diehl J.-L., Lefrant J.-Y., Prat G., Richecoeur J., Nieszkowska A., Gervais C., Baudot J., Bouadma L., and Brochard L., for the Expiratory Pressure (Express) Study Group, "Positive End-Expiratory Pressure Setting in Adults With Acute Lung Injury and Acute Respiratory Distress Syndrome: A Randomized Controlled Trial," *JAMA*, vol. 299, no. 6, pp. 646–655, Feb. 2008, doi: 10.1001/jama.299.6.646.

[6] Briel M., Meade M., Mercat A., Brower R. G., Talmor D., Walter S. D., Slutsky A. S., Pullenayegum E., Zhou Q., Cook D., Brochard L., Richard J.-C. M., Lamontagne F., Bhatnagar N., Stewart T. E., and Guyatt G., "Higher vs lower positive end-expiratory pressure in patients with acute lung injury and acute respiratory distress syndrome: systematic review and meta-analysis," *JAMA*, vol. 303, no. 9, pp. 865–873, Mar. 2010, doi: 10.1001/jama.2010.218.

[7] Kacmarek R. M., Villar J., Sulemanji D., Montiel R., Ferrando C., Blanco J., Koh Y., Soler J. A., Martínez D., Hernández M., Tucci M., Borges J. B., Lubillo S., Santos A., Araujo J. B., Amato M. B. P., Suárez-Sipmann F., and Open Lung Approach Network, "Open Lung Approach for the Acute Respiratory Distress Syndrome: A Pilot, Randomized Controlled Trial," *Crit. Care Med.*, vol. 44, no. 1, pp. 32–42, Jan. 2016, doi: 10.1097/CCM.0000000000001383.

[8] Writing Group for the Alveolar Recruitment for Acute Respiratory Distress Syndrome Trial (ART) Investigators, "Effect of Lung Recruitment and Titrated Positive End-Expiratory Pressure (PEEP) vs Low PEEP on Mortality in Patients With Acute Respiratory Distress Syndrome: A Randomized Clinical Trial," *JAMA*, vol. 318, no. 14, pp. 1335–1345, Oct. 2017, doi: 10.1001/jama.2017.14171.

[9] Hodgson C. L., Cooper D. J., Arabi Y., King V., Bersten A., Bihari S., Brickell K., Davies A., Fahey C., Fraser J., McGuinness S., Murray L., Parke R., Paul E., Tuxen D., Vallance S., Young M., and Nichol A., "Maximal Recruitment Open Lung Ventilation in Acute Respiratory Distress Syndrome (PHARLAP). A Phase II, Multicenter Randomized Controlled Clinical Trial," *Am. J. Respir. Crit. Care Med.*, vol. 200, no. 11, pp. 1363–1372, Dec. 2019, doi: 10.1164/rccm.201901-0109OC.

[10] Fan E., Del Sorbo L., Goligher E. C., Hodgson C. L., Munshi L., Walkey A. J., Adhikari N. K. J., Amato M. B. P., Branson R., Brower R. G., Ferguson N. D., Gajic O., Gattinoni L., Hess D., Mancebo J., Meade M. O., McAuley D. F., Pesenti A., Ranieri V. M., Rubenfeld G. D., Rubin E., Seckel M., Slutsky A. S., Talmor D., Thompson B. T., Wunsch H., Uleryk E., Brozek J., Brochard L. J., and American Thoracic Society, European Society of Intensive Care Medicine, and Society of Critical Care Medicine, "An Official American Thoracic Society/European Society of Intensive Care Medicine/Society of Critical Care Medicine Clinical Practice Guideline: Mechanical Ventilation in Adult Patients with Acute Respiratory Distress Syndrome," *Am. J. Respir. Crit. Care Med.*, vol. 195, no. 9, pp. 1253–1263, May 2017, doi: 10.1164/rccm.201703-0548ST.

[11] Bos L. D. J. and Ware L. B., "Acute respiratory distress syndrome: causes, pathophysiology, and phenotypes," *The Lancet*, vol. 0, no. 0, Sep. 2022, doi: 10. 1016/S0140-6736(22)01485-4.

[12] Pelosi P., Ball L., Barbas C. S. V., Bellomo R., Burns K. E. A., Einav S., Gattinoni L., Laffey J. G., Marini J. J., Myatra S. N., Schultz M. J., Teboul J. L., and Rocco P. R. M., "Personalized mechanical ventilation in acute respiratory distress syndrome," *Crit. Care*, vol. 25, no. 1, p. 250, Jul. 2021, doi: 10.1186/s13054-021-03686-3.

[13] Pierrakos C., Smit M. R., Pisani L., Paulus F., Schultz M. J., Constantin J.-M., Chiumello D., Mojoli F., Mongodi S., and Bos L. D. J., "Lung Ultrasound Assessment of Focal and Non-focal Lung Morphology in Patients With Acute Respiratory Distress Syndrome," *Front. Physiol.*, vol. 12, p. 730857, 2021, doi: 10.3389/fphys.2021.730857.

[14] Goligher E. C., Kavanagh B. P., Rubenfeld G. D., Adhikari N. K. J., Pinto R., Fan E., Brochard L. J., Granton J. T., Mercat A., Marie Richard J.-C., Chretien J.-M., Jones G. L., Cook D. J., Stewart T. E., Slutsky A. S., Meade M. O., and Ferguson N. D., "Oxygenation Response to Positive End-Expiratory Pressure Predicts Mortality in Acute Respiratory Distress Syndrome. A Secondary Analysis of the LOVS and ExPress Trials," *Am. J. Respir. Crit. Care Med.*, vol. 190, no. 1, pp. 70–76, Jul. 2014, doi: 10.1164/rccm.201404-0688OC.

[15] Dianti J., Tisminetzky M., Ferreyro B. L., Englesakis M., Del Sorbo L., Sud S., Talmor D., Ball L., Meade M., Hodgson C., Beitler J. R., Sahetya S., Nichol A., Fan E., Rochwerg B., Brochard L., Slutsky A. S., Ferguson N. D., Serpa Neto A.,

Adhikari N. K. J., Angriman F., and Goligher E. C., "Association of Positive End-Expiratory Pressure and Lung Recruitment Selection Strategies with Mortality in Acute Respiratory Distress Syndrome: A Systematic Review and Network Meta-analysis," *Am. J. Respir. Crit. Care Med.*, vol. 205, no. 11, pp. 1300–1310, Jun. 2022, doi: 10.1164/rccm.202108-1972OC.

[16] Rezoagli E. and Bellani G., "How I set up positive end-expiratory pressure: evidence- and physiology-based!," *Crit. Care*, vol. 23, no. 1, p. 412, Dec. 2019, doi: 10.1186/s13054-019-2695-z.

[17] Grieco D. L., Maggiore S. M., Bellani G., Spadaro S., Spinelli E., Tonetti T., Menga L. S., Pozzi M., Battaglini D., Di Mussi R., Bruni A., De Gaetano A., Iovino C. G., Brioni M., Mojoli F., Foti G., Volta C. A., Pelosi P., Navalesi P., Grasso S., Ranieri V. M., Antonelli M., and the IPERPEEP study group, "Individualized positive end-expiratory pressure guided by end-expiratory lung volume in early acute respiratory distress syndrome: study protocol for the multicenter, randomized IPERPEEP trial," *Trials*, vol. 23, no. 1, p. 63, Jan. 2022, doi: 10.1186/s13063-021-05993-0.

[18] Grieco D. L., Bongiovanni F., Dell'Anna A. M., and Antonelli M., "Why compliance and driving pressure may be inappropriate targets for PEEP setting during ARDS," *Crit. Care Lond. Engl.*, vol. 26, no. 1, p. 234, Aug. 2022, doi: 10.1186/s13054-022-04109-7.

[19] Baedorf Kassis E., Loring S. H., and Talmor D., "Should we titrate peep based on end-expiratory transpulmonary pressure?—yes," *Ann. Transl. Med.*, vol. 6, no. 19, p. 390, Oct. 2018, doi: 10.21037/atm.2018.06.35.

[20] Constantin J.-M., Jabaudon M., Lefrant J.-Y., Jaber S., Quenot J.-P., Langeron O., Ferrandière M., Grelon F., Seguin P., Ichai C., Veber B., Souweine B., Uberti T., Lasocki S., Legay F., Leone M., Eisenmann N., Dahyot-Fizelier C., Dupont H., Asehnoune K., Sossou A., Chanques G., Muller L., Bazin J.-E., Monsel A., Borao L., Garcier J.-M., Rouby J.-J., Pereira B., Futier E., and AZUREA Network, "Personalised mechanical ventilation tailored to lung morphology versus low positive end-expiratory pressure for patients with acute respiratory distress syndrome in France (the LIVE study): a multicentre, single-blind, randomised controlled trial," *Lancet Respir. Med.*, vol. 7, no. 10, pp. 870–880, Oct. 2019, doi: 10.1016/S2213-2600(19)30138-9.

Chapter 7

Time Course of Ventilator-Induced Lung Injury

Fernanda Ferreira Cruz[1], MD, PhD
Paolo Pelosi[2,3], MD
and Patricia R.M. Rocco[1,*], MD, PhD

[1] Laboratory of Pulmonary Investigation, Carlos Chagas Filho Institute of Biophysics, Federal University of Rio de Janeiro, Rio de Janeiro, Brazil
[2] Department of Surgical Sciences and Integrated Diagnostics (DISC), University of Genoa, Genoa, Italy
[3] Anesthesia and Intensive Care, San Martino Policlinico Hospital, IRCCS for Oncology and Neurosciences, Genoa, Italy

Abstract

Mechanical ventilation is required to support respiratory function in several lung diseases, but it may initiate or worsen lung injury, a phenomenon known as ventilator-induced lung injury (VILI). VILI usually occurs in patients with underlying lung damage (sepsis, trauma, and major surgery), when the immune system is already primed for a cascading response to mechanical lung injury.

Several mechanisms of VILI have been described: (1) inspiratory and/or expiratory stress inducing overdistension (volutrauma); (2) interfaces between collapsed or edema-filled alveoli with surrounding open alveoli, acting as stress raisers; (3) alveoli that open and close repetitively during tidal breathing (atelectrauma); and (4) peripheral airway dynamics.

---

* Corresponding Author's Email: prmrocco@biof.ufrj.br.

In: Ventilator Induced Lung Injury in Non-Invasive Ventilatory Support
Editor: Antonio M. Esquinas
ISBN: 979-8-88697-840-7

Moreover, high-stretch ventilation generates the release of inflammatory mediators from the lung, leading to systemic inflammation and distal organ injury (biotrauma). Recently, patient self-inflicted lung injury has been proposed as a potential mechanism promoting VILI. Some parameters must be adjusted to mitigate VILI, such as inspiratory stress (the respiratory system inspiratory plateau pressure [Pplat]), dynamic strain (the ratio between tidal volume and the end-expiratory lung volume, or inspiratory capacity), static strain (the end-expiratory lung volume determined by positive end-expiratory pressure [PEEP]), driving pressure (the difference between Pplat and PEEP), and mechanical power (the amount of mechanical energy imparted as a function of the respiratory rate).

Regardless of the mechanism of VILI, both the alveolar capillary membrane and extracellular matrix are injured resulting in alveolar and interstitial edema, atelectasis, hemorrhage, and formation of hyaline membranes. VILI has been studied extensively in animals and patients during invasive mechanical ventilation, but few studies have been reported during spontaneous breathing and/or noninvasive ventilatory support. In this chapter, we provide an overview of the mechanisms of VILI, focusing on the most-debated aspects of VILI in patients under spontaneous breathing and/or noninvasive ventilatory support.

Keywords: patient self-inflicted lung injury, diffuse alveolar damage, non-invasive ventilation, mechanical power, driving pressure

Introduction

A diagnosis of ventilator-induced lung injury (VILI) is generally suggested at the bedside with a high level of clinical suspicion and after excluding other differential diagnoses that could closely mimic its clinical aspects. Typically, the progression of VILI is accompanied by hypoxemia and deterioration of lung mechanics [1, 2, 3].

The most common differential diagnoses of acute hypoxemia in patients undergoing spontaneous or noninvasive mechanical ventilation that should be excluded are cardiogenic edema, infective pneumonia, and broncho aspiration [4]. Clinicians should also evaluate evidence of pneumothorax, pleural effusion, auto positive end-expiratory pressure (PEEP), venous, fat, air, or amniotic fluid embolism, acute coronary syndromes, peripheral edema, ascites, and intra-abdominal hypertension. Anamnesis should clarify any pharmacologic allergy or history of transfusion of blood components. A thorough physical examination needs to be done to rule out new-onset crackles or bronchospasms, and other typical signs of all these other conditions [4]. Ventilatory settings must be carefully cross-checked to identify any possible contributing factors for acute lung injury.

Complementary examinations should be done to exclude other associated causes of hypoxemia in spontaneous breathing with and without noninvasive respiratory support. A detailed clinical evaluation at the bedside, radiologic examinations of the thoracic region (chest radiographs or computerized tomography [CT]), laboratory examinations, ultrasonography of the chest and abdomen, diaphragmatic echocardiography along with cardiovascular evaluation with electrocardiogram (ECG) and echocardiogram can help to rule out most of the above causes [4, 5]. Auto PEEP can be detected by expiratory port occlusion at the end of the set exhalation period. Radiologic findings in VILI resemble acute respiratory distress syndrome [6]. Chest radiographs may show diffuse alveolar/interstitial infiltrates in both lungs without cardiac enlargement, whereas chest CT images may present heterogeneous atelectasis and consolidation with focal areas of hyperlucency suggestive of alveolar overdistension [6].

Laboratory investigations include cardiac enzymes, levels of lipase, culture of blood and other body fluids. Lower limb doppler ultrasonography and CT pulmonary angiography may be required in certain cases. Bronchoscopy and biopsy are rarely indicated.

In this chapter, we provide an overview of the mechanisms of VILI focusing on the most-debated aspects of VILI in patients under spontaneous breathing and/or noninvasive ventilatory support.

Mechanisms of VILI

Several mechanisms of VILI have been described: (1) inspiratory and/or expiratory stress inducing overdistension (volutrauma); (2) interfaces between collapsed or edema-filled alveoli with surrounding open alveoli, acting as stress raisers; (3) alveoli that open and close repetitively during tidal breathing (atelectrauma); and (4) peripheral airway dynamics. Moreover, high-stretch ventilation generates the release of inflammatory mediators from the lung, leading to systemic inflammation and distal organ injury (biotrauma). Recently, patient self-inflicted lung injury (P-SILI) has been proposed as a potential mechanism promoting VILI [1].

Some parameters must be adjusted to mitigate VILI, such as inspiratory stress (the respiratory system inspiratory plateau pressure [Pplat]); dynamic strain (the ratio between tidal volume and the end-expiratory lung volume, or inspiratory capacity); static strain (the end-expiratory lung volume determined by PEEP); driving pressure (the difference between Pplat and PEEP); and mechanical power, (the amount of mechanical energy imparted as a function of the respiratory rate).

Mechanical Power

To date, most studies have focused on measurement of mechanical power during volume-controlled ventilation, but further studies are required to evaluate its measurement during noninvasive ventilation. Mechanical power can be computed according to parameters set by the clinician at the bedside: tidal volume (V_T), airway pressure (Paw), inspiratory airflow (V'), PEEP, respiratory rate, and other individual variables such as peak, plateau and driving pressures [7]. Gattinoni et al., [8] have proposed simple ventilator software for the mechanical power equation (hence identifying the contribution of each component causing VILI) to easily compute and analyse at the bedside.

Currently, three different mathematical equations are available to calculate mechanical power during volume-controlled ventilation, from pressure–volume (P/V) curves to more complex formulas that consider both dynamic (kinetic) and static (potential) components; simpler methods mainly consider the dynamic component. The first method is based on an analysis of quasi-static P/V curves of the respiratory system. Under low-flow conditions, the influence of the resistive properties will be reduced, and the elastic properties of the respiratory system will be the main component of the mechanical energy calculation. The total area of the rectangle, obtained by the product of the volume difference (ΔV) by the pressure difference (ΔP), should be calculated. The area under the curve can be calculated as the integral of the pressure with respect to volume. The difference between the total area of the rectangle and the area under the curve corresponds to energy transfer (ml cmH_2O or Joules). This value (energy), multiplied by the respiratory rate, gives the mechanical power. Using this method, the potential energy generating static strain in the respiratory system (PEEP) is not considered.

There is a second method that includes both the resistive properties (apparatus/airways and tissue resistance) and the variation in lung volume corresponding to the PEEP level. The third method for calculating mechanical power uses the end-of-inspiration occlusion method. This calculation is considered a simplification of the second method. It computes the most important component, the driving mechanical power. This method does not consider the PEEP level or the resistive component (Figure 1) [7, 8]. The net effect of increasing the PEEP level in terms of outcomes during ventilatory support may depend on its ability to increase the lung surface area, which will decrease the excursion of tidal pressure and the mechanical energy transfer from ventilator to lung [1, 9, 10].

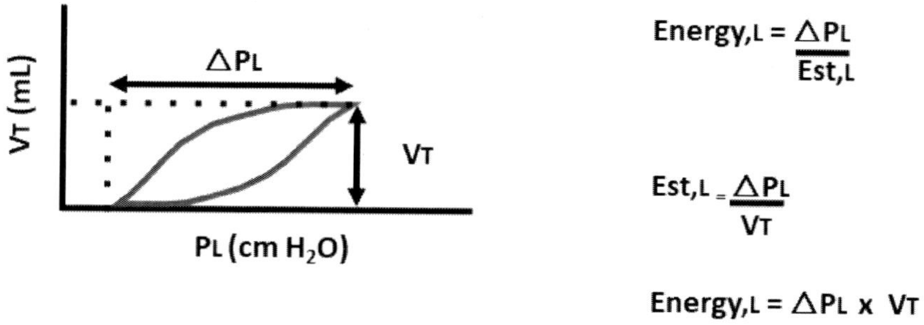

Figure 1. Representative volume-PL curve. V_T, tidal volume; ΔP_L, transpulmonary driving pressure; EstL, static lung elastance. Mechanical energy (EnergyL) was calculated based on the equation described by Guerin et al. [19] and the simplified formula of Marini and Jaber [9] as $Energy_L = \Delta P_L^2/EstL = \Delta P_L^2/(\Delta P_L/V_T) = \Delta P_L \times V_T$, which is the area of the rectangle. Therefore, one must compute the area of the rectangle and divide the result by two. This simplified equation estimates elastic work without considering resistive properties and PEEP.

Mechanical power should be normalized to the amount of pulmonary surface ventilated; the ratio of mechanical power to the alveolar area exposed to energy delivery is called the intensity. For a given mechanical power, the intensity is higher in lungs with fewer ventilated areas, and at the interface between lung zones with different mechanical properties. If the lung surface that can accommodate the mechanical power transfer is large, VILI is less likely to occur. On the other hand, if the lung surface is small, VILI is more likely to develop for the same mechanical power delivered. In progression of VILI, not only the lung surface but also the open/closed interfaces are important; they have been associated with high inflammation, increasing proportionally with the severity of the lung condition [1, 9].

Inspiratory Effort

Vigorous spontaneous breathing efforts during noninvasive respiratory support in patients with severe lung injury can worsen lung injury [11]. Reliable evaluation of the inspiratory effort can be achieved by assessing the esophageal pressure (Pes) signal as an estimation of the pleural pressure using an esophageal catheter. Transpulmonary pressure (P_L), the difference between alveolar pressure and Pes, is the distending pressure of the lung and reflects the inspiratory effort. In lung diseases, greater inspiratory efforts are required to obtain a similar tidal volume, and early spontaneous breathing effort yields higher negative pleural pressure and P_L. Airway occlusion pressure at 100 ms (P0.1) has been used to estimate the inspiratory effort and has shown good correlation with the work of breathing and pressure–time product) [12].

The esophageal pressure inspiratory swing (ΔPes) is much easier to measure at the bedside and can be monitored directly on some ventilator screens. Recording ΔPes allows detection of inappropriate inspiratory efforts. When the absolute value of ΔPes is lower than 2–3 cm H_2O, it is commonly understood as a sign of overassistance. On the other side, an absolute value of ΔPes higher than 8–12 cmH_2O is considered as a marker of underassistance [13]. However, the use of Pes in the clinical setting remains limited because it is often viewed as a research tool dedicated to expert centers. The electrical activity of the diaphragm (EAdi) can be measured using a specific esogastric tube and a dedicated ventilator. EAdi is a surrogate of respiratory drive and is closely correlated with respiratory effort indices. Ultrasonography of the diaphragm can also be used to assess patient–ventilator interactions and quantify the thickening fraction, which correlates with inspiratory effort.

Esophageal manometry is not easy to implement at the bedside in all clinical cases, especially in unstable patients with respiratory failure and severe impairment of gas exchange, therefore an easy way to perform respiratory monitoring of inspiratory effort in patients with acute respiratory failure would be useful in all patients at risk of P-SILI. In this context, recent findings have shown that nasal pressure swings can be used at the bedside during noninvasive respiratory support, because nasal pressure swing was found to be highly correlated with esophageal pressure swing in these patients [14, 15].

Mechanisms of P-SILI

In injured lungs during noninvasive respiratory support, the mechanisms underlying P-SILI may be associated with (1) increased global and regional strain in normal aerated lungs for the same tidal volume, thus leading to changes in diaphragm function and morphology; (2) increased lung stress; (3) inhomogeneous distribution of ventilation increased inspiratory effort may yield more negative pleural swings and *(pendelluft* phenomena); (4) changes in lung perfusion (inspiratory effort may compress pulmonary capillary vessels, thus increasing the pulmonary resistance); and (5) patient–ventilator asynchronies [13].

How to Reduce the Risk of P-SILI during Noninvasive Respiratory Support

Daily analysis of clinical data and ventilator waveforms should be performed to detect situations at risk of P-SILI, especially when esophageal pressure monitoring and respiratory effort measurement are not routinely performed. The following parameters need to be evaluated: work of breathing, level of sedation and consciousness, hemodynamic parameters, and gas exchange.

Three strategies have been suggested to minimize P-SILI:

(a) Limitation of V_T, even though V_T monitoring is not easy at the bedside when using high flow nasal cannula oxygen therapy (HFNOT) or continuous positive airway pressure (CPAP) via helmet,
(b) The application of PEEP, which may reduce atelectasis, distal airway collapse, regional overdistension, *pendelluft*, diaphragm damage, and
(c) Reduction of spontaneous effort.

All three of these strategies should be combined with appropriate sedation and metabolic control. To date, no clinical study has demonstrated whether these strategies may limit the risk of P-SILI and improve patient outcomes.

Non-invasive Respiratory Support

Non-invasive positive pressure ventilation (NPPV) is the first step in acute respiratory failure. The mortality rate after 90 days was lower among patients on HFNOT compared with those on NPPV [13]. The ROX index has been used to help recognize the patients at risk of HFNOT failure. The ROX index is defined as the ratio of peripheral oxygen saturation (Spo_2)/fraction of inspired oxygen (Fio_2) to the respiratory rate, i.e., a ratio of the severity of hypoxemia to a surrogate of respiratory drive [13]. Failure of HFNOT can be predicted when the ROX index is lower than 2.85, 3.47, and 3.85 at 2, 6, and 12 h after initiation, respectively.

Different interfaces have been proposed to deliver CPAP, such as facemask and helmet CPAP. The use of a helmet may offer extra protection against P-SILI. When comparing HFNOT and helmet CPAP in patients with moderate to severe hypoxemia, helmet CPAP reduced inspiratory effort with similar transpulmonary pressure swings, $Paco_2$, and comfort. Further studies are required to evaluate the best noninvasive respiratory support strategy in patients with acute respiratory failure associated with reduced risk of P-SILI and better prognosis.

Conclusion

The mechanisms of VILI described here include volutrauma, atelectrauma, and biotrauma. To prevent VILI, mechanical ventilation strategies should minimize inspiratory/expiratory stress, static/dynamic strain, mechanical power, and intensity, as well as mitigate the hemodynamic consequences of noninvasive respiratory support. In injured lungs, during noninvasive respiratory support, P-SILI may occur due to increased effort and thus transpulmonary driving pressure, *pendelluft* phenomena, changes in lung perfusion, and patient–ventilator asynchronies.

There are controversies regarding the mechanisms of P-SILI. Clinical signs of worsening hypoxia despite the beginning of noninvasive ventilation can suggest VILI.

References

[1] Silva P L, Ball L, Rocco P R M, Pelosi P. Physiological and pathophysiological consequences of mechanical ventilation. Semin. *Respir. Crit. Care Med.* 2022; 43: 321–334. doi: 10.1055/s-0042-1744447.

[2] Rocco P R M, Silva P L, Samary C S, Hayat Syed M K, Marini J J. Elastic power but not driving power is the key promoter of ventilator-induced lung injury in experimental acute respiratory distress syndrome. *Crit. Care*. 2020; 24: 284. doi: 10.1186/s13054-020-03011-4.

[3] Marini J J, Rocco P R M, Gattinoni L. Static and dynamic contributors to ventilator-induced lung injury in clinical practice. pressure, energy, and power. *Am. J. Respir. Crit. Care. Med.* 2020; 201: 767–774. doi: 10.1164/rccm.201908-1545CI.

[4] Kumar A K A, Anjum F. *Ventilator-Induced Lung Injury (VILI)* [Updated 2022 Jun 19]. In: StatPearls [Internet]. Treasure Island (FL): StatPearls Publishing; 2022. Available from: https://www.ncbi.nlm.nih.gov/books/NBK563244/.

[5] Robba Chiara , Adrian Wong, Daniele Poole, Ashraf Al Tayar, Robert T Arntfield, Michelle S Chew, Francesco Corradi, Ghislaine Douflé, Alberto Goffi, Massimo Lamperti· Paul Mayo, Antonio Messina, Silvia Mongodi, Mangala Narasimhan, Corina Puppo, Aarti Sarwal, Michel Slama, Fabio S Taccone, Philippe Vignon, Antoine Vieillard-Baron, European Society of Intensive Care Medicine task force for critical care ultrasonography. Basic ultrasound head-to-toe skills for intensivists in the general and neuro intensive care unit population: consensus and expert recommendations of the European Society of Intensive Care Medicine. *Intensive Care Med*. 2021; 47: 1347–1367. doi: 10.1007/s00134-021-06486-z.

[6] Chiurazzi C, M Gotti, M Amini, C Rovati, I Algieri, M Brioni, A Cammaroto, C Bacile di Castiglione, K Nikolla, C Montaruli, S Luoni, B Comini, G Rossignoli, G Conte, T Langer, M Cressoni, and L Gattinoni. Time course of VILI development: a CT scan study. *Intensive Care Med. Exp*. 2014; 2(Suppl 1): O20. doi: 10.1186/2197-425X-2-S1-O20.

[7] Silva P L, Ball L, Rocco PRM, Pelosi P. Power to mechanical power to minimize ventilator-induced lung injury? *Intensive Care Med. Exp*. 2019; 7(Suppl 1): 38. doi: 10.1186/s40635-019-0243-4.

[8] Gattinoni L, Tonetti T, Cressoni M, Cadringher P, Herrmann P, Moerer O, Protti A, Gotti M, Chiurazzi C, Carlesso E, Chiumello D, Quintel M. Ventilator-related causes of lung injury: the mechanical power. *Intensive Care Med*. 2016; 42: 1567–1575. doi: 10.1007/s00134-016-4505-2.

[9] Silva P L, Pelosi P, Rocco P R M. Understanding the mysteries of mechanical power. *Anesthesiology*. 2020; 132: 949–950. doi: 10.1097/ALN.0000000000003222.

[10] Pelosi Paolo , Lorenzo Ball, Carmen S V Barbas, Rinaldo Bellomo, Karen E A Burns, Sharon Einav, Luciano Gattinoni, John G Laffey, John J Marini, Sheila N Myatra, Marcus J Schultz, Jean Louis Teboul, Patricia R M Rocco. Personalized mechanical ventilation in acute respiratory distress syndrome. *Crit. Care*. 2021; 25: 250. doi: 10.1186/s13054-021-03686-3.

[11] Brochard L, Slutsky A, Pesenti A. Mechanical ventilation to minimize progression of lung injury in acute respiratory failure. *Am. J. Respir. Crit. Care Med.* 2017; 195: 438–442. doi: 10.1164/rccm.201605-1081CP.

[12] Foti G, Cereda M, Banfi G, Pelosi P, Fumagalli R, Pesenti A. End-inspiratory airway occlusion: a method to assess the pressure developed by inspiratory muscles in patients with acute lung injury undergoing pressure support. *Am. J. Respir. Crit. Care Med.* 1997; 156(4 Pt 1): 1210–1216. doi: 10.1164/ajrccm.156.4.96-02031.

[13] Carteaux G, Parfait M, Combet M, Haudebourg AF, Tuffet S, Mekontso Dessap A. Patient-self-inflicted lung injury: a practical review. *J. Clin. Med.* 2021; 10: 2738. doi: 10.3390/jcm10122738.

[14] Tonelli R, Cortegiani A, Marchioni A, Fantini R, Tabbì L, Castaniere I, Biagioni E, Busani S, Nani C, Cerbone C, Vermi M, Gozzi F, Bruzzi G, Manicardi L, Pellegrino MR, Beghè B, Girardis M, Pelosi P, Gregoretti C, Ball L, Clini E. Nasal pressure swings as the measure of inspiratory effort in spontaneously breathing patients with de novo acute respiratory failure. *Crit. Care.* 2022; 26: 70. doi: 10.1186/s13054-022-03938-w.

[15] Pelosi Paolo, Roberto Tonelli, Chiara Torregiani, Elisa Baratella, Marco Confalonieri, Denise Battaglini, Alessandro Marchioni, Paola Confalonieri, Enrico Clini, Francesco Salton, Barbara Ruaro. Different methods to improve the monitoring of noninvasive respiratory support of patients with severe pneumonia/ARDS due to COVID-19: an update. *J. Clin. Med.* 2022; 11: 1704. doi: 10.3390/jcm11061704.

Chapter 8

Hyperoxic Acute Lung Injury: Pathophysiology

Martina Flora*, **MD**
Anna Annunziata, MD
Lidia Atripaldi, MD
and Giuseppe Fiorentino, MD
Division of Respiratory Physiopathology and Rehabilitation,
A.O.R.N. "Dei Colli" - Monaldi Hospital, Naples, Italy

Abstract

Oxygen therapy is useful in the treatment of hypoxemia and oxygen supplementation is widely used in various clinical conditions. Even if the life treating effects of the oxygen are well known, the toxicity is usually less considered. Hyperoxia induces oxidative stress and systemic inflammation, leading to histopathological modifications similar to acute respiratory distress syndrome (ARDS).

Several studies found an association between excessive use of oxygen and poor outcome in different clinical settings. The conservative oxygen therapy was proposed with the intention of minimizing oxygen toxicity in critically ill patients, but studies showed contradictory findings. In this chapter, we want to report the possible acute and chronic oxygen toxicity and review the recent evidence on the outcome of different oxygen supplementation strategies in critical care settings.

Keywords: hyperoxia acute lung injury, hyperoxia, oxygen therapy, conservative oxygen therapy, oxygen toxicity

---

* Corresponding Author's Email: martinafloraa@gmail.com.

In: Ventilator Induced Lung Injury in Non-Invasive Ventilatory Support
Editor: Antonio M. Esquinas
ISBN: 979-8-88697-840-7

Introduction

Oxygen is widely used in the treatment of critically ill patients in various clinical settings. It is routinely administered with some benefits during cardiopulmonary resuscitation from cardiac arrest, stroke, and traumatic brain injury. In fact, various guidelines encourage the use of supplemental oxygen in medical emergencies. Moreover, due to different causes, oxygen supplementation represents one of the first line treatments for hypoxemia, as well as a cornerstone of the treatment of acute respiratory distress syndrome (ARDS) and mechanically ventilated patients. Even if the life treating effects of the oxygen are well known, sometimes the risks of excessive oxygen administration are less taken into account by healthcare workers [1, 2].

Negative consequences of oxygen have been known for about a century. In 1899, James Lorrain Smith observed that mice exposed to FiO_2 0.7-0.8 died of respiratory failure. Later, studies on both animals and humans confirmed the evidence about the acute pulmonary toxicity induced by a high concentration or prolonged oxygen exposure, the so-called "Hyperoxic Acute Lung Injury" (HALI). Hyperoxia enhances oxidative stress and inflammatory response, leading to alveolar collapse, alveolar-capillary barrier injury, surfactant dysfunction and impairment in mucociliary clearance. Pulmonary consequences consist of pulmonary edema, adsorptive and obstructive atelectasis, reduction in lung compliance and increased risk of infection. Finally, lung involvement can progress in fibrosis and emphysema. In addition to this, it must be underlined that hyperoxia may also have systemic effects such as cardiovascular and neurological consequences. The impaired coronary perfusion, reducing cardiac output and increasing peripheral vascular resistances, may exacerbate the hemodynamics status of hypoxemic critical patients [3, 4].

Respiratory symptoms in the early phase consist of bronchial irritation, cough, sore throat, tracheobronchitis and substernal pain. However, with the progression of lung injury and gas exchange impairment, clinical manifestations are similar to the "acute lung injury" triggered by other causes, with progressive hypoxia, dyspnea and tachypnea. Therefore, in patients with severe respiratory failure, it is very difficult to recognize whether the deterioration of lung function is due either to the progression of the disease or to some oxygen toxicity. In fact, also pathological changes mimic Diffuse Alveolar Damage of ARDS with evidence of alveolar injury, fibrin thrombi and hyaline membrane. The manifestations of hyperoxia are dose, time and age dependent, despite a unique threshold, still on debate. Data suggested that already a ventilation with $FiO_2 > 0.5$ for prolonged time was able to enhance lung toxicity. Furthermore, oxygen treatment with FiO_2 from 0.8 to 0.1 for 3-5 days induced destruction of the alveolar capillary endothelium in animals. In summary, in different animal models, an exposure of oxygen with FiO_2 varying from 0.4 to 0.1 was associated with typical histopathological characteristics of hyperoxia. These effects were found both in the early phase (i.e., within 90 minutes of exposure) and in the late one (i.e., after 8 weeks) [5].

Evidence from Clinical Studies

Clinical evidence has supported the preclinical data of oxygen toxicity and, in several observational studies in ICU patients, the association between hyperoxia and mortality was found. De Jonge et al., in a large retrospective study of ICU patients, showed a relationship between mortality and FiO_2 in a linear mode. In addition, a U-shaped relationship between PaO_2 and mortality was established. They stated the highest mortality with both low PaO_2 and high PaO_2 in the first 24 hours [6].

A systematic review and meta-analysis reported increasing mortality in ICU patients with stroke, traumatic brain injury and post cardiac arrest treated with high oxygen concentrations [2]. On the contrary, other studies did not confirm these data. Eastwood et al., in an observational study of 150,000 patients, underlined that hyperoxia was common in the early ICU admission but they did not find its association with an increased risk of mortality [7]. Hence, it is probable that these contradictory proofs might be due to the large study heterogeneity. In fact, the observational studies use very different cuts off to define hyperoxemia with a spectrum of PaO_2 value from 300 to 120 mmHg. Moreover, heterogeneous measures were analyzed and most of data were evaluated in the first 24 hours of ICU-admission [4]. Handrik et al., in an observational study, evidenced that the association between hypoxemia and mortality depended on the oxygenation metric used. As the authors showed, the metric of central tendencies (average and medial PaO_2) had a strong relationship with outcomes [8].

The harmful effects of oxygen are particularly worrying in critical patients affected by acute respiratory distress syndrome (ARDS) and mechanically ventilated patients. In particular, the subset of patients with severe ARDS requires prolonged exposure to high oxygen concentration which increases the risk of HALI, especially in some clinical contests such as viral pneumonia and hypermetabolic state (sepsis and trauma). Additionally, ARDS patients usually need to be mechanically ventilated, and this exposes them to the risk of Ventilator Induced Lung Injury (VILI).

Several evidence focused on the potential synergistic or additive effects of high tidal volume (Vt) ventilator strategy and hyperoxia to amplify VILI. In animal model of ventilation with high-stretch Vt, the combination or the pre-treatment with high oxygen concentration enhanced the severity of ventilator-induced lung injury (VILI) and pathological results. In fact, these effects were observed in the group with high-stretch Vt with ambient FiO_2, in the group with low Vt with high FiO_2 (FiO_2 0.8-1), as well as in the group with high Vt and FiO_2. To explain the possible origins of this synergistic effect, an *in vitro* study found that both hyperoxemia and mechanical stress caused remodeling and modification of epithelial cells cytoskeleton, that became stiffened and more sensitive on developing a stretch-induced injury. Furthermore, ventilation in overdistended region caused lung injury and, probably, hyperinflation with high oxygen concentration may have enhanced this damage [9].

In order to minimize the detrimental effects of oxygen supplementation in these patients, a conservative strategy in oxygen therapy was proposed. It means that the concentration of oxygen administered to the patients was titrated to achieve an oxygenation (measured as PaO_2 or SpO_2) that was consider acceptable with the aim of balancing useful and toxic effects of oxygen therapy.

In 2016, Giradis et al., realized the first randomized clinical trial, comparing the effects of the two different supplemental oxygen strategies on mortality in critically ill patients. The conservative group with target SpO_2 of 94-98% reported improved outcomes, demonstrating lower mortality and less event of shock, liver failure and bacteremia [10]. Therefore, many studies compared conservative versus conventional oxygen therapy in acute illness with contradictory results (See Table 1).

In a meta-analysis of 25 RTC and 16037 patients affected by sepsis, stroke, trauma, myocardial infraction and cardiac arrest, Chung et al., showed that liberal oxygen strategy (median FiO_2 0.52, IQR 0.28-1.0) increased short and long-term mortality in comparison with the conservative strategy (median FiO_2 0.21, IQR 0.21-0.25) [11].

On the contrary, more recent studies did not confirm the superiority of conservative oxygen strategy in term of clinical outcomes (See Table 1).

Table 1. Comparison between conservative versus conventional oxygen therapy strategies in recent studies of ICU patients

Reference	Country	Study design	Diagnosis	Sample size	Conservative Group definition	Findings in conservative O2 therapy group vs conventional O2 group
Suzuki et al., 2014	Australia	Single center pilot prospective before-after.	Cardiovascular, gastrointestinal, neurological, respiratory diseases, sepsis, others.	105	SpO2 90-92%	Safety. Trend in decreasing risk of non-respiratory organ failure and lactate level.
Suzuki et al., 2015	Australia	Single center pilot prospective before-after.	Cardiovascular, gastrointestinal, neurological, respiratory diseases, sepsis, other.	105	SpO2 90-92%	Lower atelectasis score. More ventilator-free days.
Helmerhorst et al., 2016	Netherlands	Multi-center before-after.	Medical.	15045	PaO2 55-86 mmHg SpO2 90-95%	Safety and feasibility. Lower hospital mortality. More ventilator-free days.
Girardis et al., OXYGEN-ICU trial, 2016	Italy	Single-center open label RCT.	Medical, surgical.	434	SpO2 94-98%	Lower ICU mortality. Lower incidence of new infection and shock.
Panwar et al., CLOSE trial, 2016	Australia, New Zealand, France	Pilot multi-center RCT.	Trauma, medical, surgical.	103	SpO2 88-92%	No difference in 90-day mortality and new organ dysfunction. A trend of lower mortality (in respiratory subgroup analysis).

Table 1. (Continued)

Reference	Country	Study design	Diagnosis	Sample size	Conservative Group definition	Findings in conservative O2 therapy group vs conventional O2 group
Eastwood et al., 2016	Australia	Retrospective nested cohort study.	Cardiac arrest.	100	SpO_2 88-92%	Safety and feasibility. Shorter ICU length of stay.
Eastwood et al., 2019	Australia	Uncontrolled before-and-after study.	Cardiac surgery.	543	SpO_2 88-92%	Safety and feasibility. No differences in 30-days mortality and ICU length of stay.
Mackle et al., ICU-ROX trial, 2020	Australia, New Zealand	Multi-center RCT.	Surgery, ARDS, acute brain disease. Suspected hypoxic-ischemic encephalopathy.	965	SpO_2 90-97% FiO_2 as low as possible	No differences in number of ventilator-free days, 90-day and 180-day mortality.
Barrot et al., LOCO2 trial, 2020	France	Prospective multi-center RCT.	ARDS	201	PaO_2 55-70 mmHg SpO_2 88-92%	No differences in 28-days mortality. A trend of increased mortality at 90 days and mesenteric ischemia.
Schjørring et al., HOT-ICU trial, 2021	Denmark, Switzerland, Finland, Netherlands, Norway, UK, Iceland	Multi-center RCT.	Pneumonia, trauma, stroke, brain injury, myocardial infarction, intestinal ischemia, cardiac arrest, ARDS.	2888	PaO_2 60 mmHg	No differences in 90-days mortality, percentage of days alive without life support, percentage of days alive after hospital discharge, and serious adverse events.

In the prospective randomized $LOCO_2$ trial, the authors compared the treatment with conservative oxygen versus liberal oxygen strategy in ARDS mechanically ventilated patients, targeting respectively PaO_2 55-70 mmHg SpO_2 88-92% and PaO_2 90-105 mmHg $SpO_2 \geq 96\%$. They found that the conservative oxygen protocol did not reduce 28-days mortality. They even showed a non-significant lower 90 day-mortality in conventional oxygen group and five mesenteric ischemic events in conservative oxygen group. In fact, the trial was early closed for safety reasons. The evidence seems to be in contrast with previous studies (See Table 1), but in the latter trial mentioned, the severity of ARDS was higher than in the others, with more than 40% of patients with $PaO_2/FiO_2 < 100$. Furthermore, oxygen values that defined the conservative oxygen group were lower than those used in other trials and the ones considered by some guidelines on ARDS. Hence, it is possible that patients treated with conservative oxygen in this study may have been exposed to the risk of hypoxemia [12].

Recently, a meta-analysis of nine studies published from 2014 to 2021 has analyzed 5,759 patients hospitalized in the ICU and the outcomes were as follows: mortality, length of ICU and hospital stay, new infections. In this study, no superiority of conservative oxygen therapy has been shown with respect to the conventional one. At the same time, the authors found that conservative oxygen therapy reduced the length of mechanical ventilation and new organ failure [13].

The different results of the studies on mortality might be due to several factors. First, the different clinical conditions of patients such as sepsis, ARDS, cardiac arrest, and hypoxic-ischemic encephalopathy might have had different impacts on the response to conservative oxygen therapy. Moreover, the severity of the patients enrolled was not homogeneous. Then, as shown in Table 1, the definition of "conservative oxygen therapy" and the outcome explored were very different among the studies.

The evidence on the use of oxygen therapy in various clinical settings remains contradictory and lacks high quality. In addition, many guidelines do not clearly indicate a safe upper limit of oxygen supplementation. Even if studies identified a linear association between PaO_2 and mortality, they did not find a unique threshold of safe PaO_2. Likewise, a recent systematic review failed to identify a safe threshold of oxygen exposure, probably due to heterogeneity of the studies in the definition of endpoints and both low and high FiO_2. Authors only suggested keeping FiO_2 under 0.8 to minimize the risk of atelectasis occurrence [14].

Long-term Oxygen Therapy in Chronic Lung Disease

Even if there is different evidence of oxygen toxicity in acute settings, little is known about the effects of long-term O_2 therapy in chronic lung diseases. Patients with chronic respiratory failure due to chronic obstructive pulmonary disease (COPD) or diffuse parenchymal lung disease have to undergo a long period of oxygen therapy. In 1970s, Petty et al., showed classical findings of hyperoxia on the autopsy of a half of COPD patients in long-term oxygen therapy, with FiO_2 near 0.22-0.27. Moreover, more recent studies underlined that also short-term oxygen treatment of 18-48 hours produced oxidative stress in COPD patients. However, in these patients the oxidative stress may have multifactorial geneses such as smoking and infective exacerbations [3].

Conclusion

The harmful acute and chronic effects of oxygen are documented in preclinical and clinical studies, and they must be considered by clinicians when they administer oxygen therapy. Unfortunately, little is still known about a threshold for oxygen toxicity in terms of concentration and duration of exposition. Moreover, it is not even clear which is the safe limit value of oxygenation to titrate oxygen supplementation in critical care patients. Therefore, even if there are not specific guidelines, it is prudent to promote a careful use of oxygen supplementation in critical care units, in order to balance positive and negative effects of oxygen therapy.

References

[1] de Graaff, Dongelmans, Binnekade, de Jonge E. 2011. "Clinicians' response to hyperoxia in ventilated patients in a Dutch ICU depends on the level of FiO2." *Intensive Care Medicine* 37(1):46-51. doi:10.1007/s00134-010-2025-z.

[2] Damiani, Adrario, Girardis, Romano, Pelaia, Singer, Donati A. 2014. "Arterial hyperoxia and mortality in critically ill patients: a systematic review and meta-analysis." *Critical Care* 18(6):711. doi:10.1186/s13054-014-0711-x.

[3] Kallet, Matthay A. Matthay. 2013. "Hyperoxic acute lung injury." *Respiratory Care 58*(1), 123–141. doi:10.4187/respcare.01963.

[4] Damiani, E., Donati, A., & Girardis, M. 2018. "Oxygen in the critically ill: friend or foe?" *Current Opinion in Anaesthesiology 31*(2):129–135. doi:10.1097/ACO.0000 000000000559.

[5] Pannu R. Sonal. 2016. "Too Much Oxygen: Hyperoxia and Oxygen Management in Mechanically Ventilated Patients." *Seminars in Respiratory and Critical Care Medicine 37*(1):16–22. doi:10.1055/s-0035-1570359.

[6] de Jonge, Peelen, Keijzers, Joore, de Lange, van der Voort, Bosman, de Waal, Wesselink, de Keizer F. Nicolette. 2008. "Association between administered oxygen, arterial partial oxygen pressure and mortality in mechanically ventilated intensive care unit patients." *Critical Care* 12(6):R156. doi:10.1186/cc7150.

[7] Eastwood, Bellomo, Bailey, Taori, Pilcher, Young, Beasley R. 2012. "Arterial oxygen tension and mortality in mechanically ventilated patients." *Intensive Care Medicine* 38(1):91-98. doi:10.1007/s00134-011-2419-6.

[8] Helmerhorst, Schultz, van der Voort, Bosman, Juffermans, de Wilde, van den Akker-van Marle, van Bodegom-Vos, de Vries, Eslami, de Keizer, Abu-Hanna, van Westerloo, de Jonge E. 2016. "Effectiveness and Clinical Outcomes of a Two-Step Implementation of Conservative Oxygenation Targets in Critically Ill Patients: A Before and After Trial." *Critical Care Medicine* 44(3):554-563. doi:10.1097/CCM.0000000000001461.

[9] Kellet, Branson D. Richard. 2016. "Should Oxygen Therapy Be Tightly Regulated to Minimize Hyperoxia in Critically Ill Patients?" *Respiratory Care* 61(6):801-817. doi:10.4187/respcare.04933.

[10] Girardis, Busani, Damiani, Donati, Rinaldi, Marudi, Morelli, Antonelli, Singer M. 2016. "Effect of Conservative vs Conventional Oxygen Therapy on Mortality Among Patients in an Intensive Care Unit: The Oxygen-ICU Randomized Clinical Trial." *JAMA* 316(15):1583-1589. doi:10.1001/jama.2016.11993.

[11] Chu, Kim, Young, Zamiri, Almenawer, Jaeschke, Szczeklik, Schünemann, Neary, Alhazzani W. 2018. "Mortality and morbidity in acutely ill adults treated with liberal versus conservative oxygen therapy (IOTA): a systematic review and meta-analysis." *Lancet* 391(10131):1693-1705. doi:10.1016/S0140-6736(18) 304 79-3.

[12] Barrot, Asfar, Mauny, Winiszewski, Montini, Badie, Quenot, Pili-Floury, Bouhemad, Louis, Souweine, Collange, Pottecher, Levy, Puyraveau, Vettoretti, Constantin, Capellier G.; LOCO2 Investigators and REVA Research Network. 2020. "Liberal or Conservative Oxygen Therapy for Acute Respiratory Distress Syndrome." *The New England Journal of Medicine* 382(11):999-1008. doi:10.1056/NEJMoa1916431.

[13] Ni, Luo, Yu, Liu, Liang, Liang A. Zong. 2018. "The effect of high-flow nasal cannula in reducing the mortality and the rate of endotracheal intubation when used before mechanical ventilation compared with conventional oxygen therapy and noninvasive positive pressure ventilation. A systematic review and meta-analysis." *The American Journal of Emergency Medicine* 36(2):226-233. doi: 10.1016/j.ajem.2017.07.083.

[14] Lassen, Risgaard, Baekgaard, Rasmussen S. Lars. 2021. "Determining a safe upper limit of oxygen supplementation for adult patients: a systematic review." *BMJ Open.* 11(7):e045057. Published 2021 Jul 26. doi:10.1136/bmjopen-2020-045057.

Chapter 9

Ventilatory Approaches and High-Flow Nasal Cannula: Clinical Implications

Dimitrios A. Lagonidis*, **MD, PhD**
Intensive Care Unit German Oncologic Center, Limassol, Cyprus

Abstract

The role of spontaneous breathing in patients with acute hypoxemic respiratory failure (AHRF) and acute respiratory distress syndrome (ARDS) is not clear. High-flow nasal cannula (HFNC) and other non-invasive respiratory support modalities [e.g., continuous positive airway pressure (CPAP) and mask- or helmet- non-invasive positive pressure ventilation (NPPV)] may reduce intubation rates, by improving oxygenation and by protecting the lung and the diaphragm. However, treatment failure is associated with increased mortality due to delayed intubation.

The vicious circle deriving from hypoxemia, increased respiratory drive, abnormal respiratory mechanics, and inhomogeneous lung inflation, comprises the fundamental mechanism of the potential harmful effects that can arise during spontaneous breathing in patients suffering from ARDS. Recently patient self-inflicted lung injury (P-SILI) has been suggested as a mechanism for deteriorating lung injury in ARDS patients.

Spontaneous breathing has the risk that vigorous inspiratory effort:

a) Generates high regional transpulmonary pressures, shifting gas from the non-dependent to dependent lung zones (i.e., pendelluft) and creating high dorsal tidal volume and cyclic opening/closing of the dependent regions further worsening the lung injury (atelectrauma);

* Corresponding Author's Email: lagonidis@gmail.com.

In: Ventilator Induced Lung Injury in Non-Invasive Ventilatory Support
Editor: Antonio M. Esquinas
ISBN: 979-8-88697-840-7

b) Results in the inflation of high tidal volume in lung regions with compromised aerated areas causing local over-stretch and additional lung damage (i.e., P-SILI);
c) Creates abnormal increases in transvascular pressures in pulmonary circulation yielding negative pressure pulmonary edema;
d) Promotes diaphragmatic injury.

Not all AHRF patients are at risk of developing P-SILI. Those with PaO_2/FiO_2 < 200 mmHg may constitute the most vulnerable sub-population. Current conditional guidelines suggest HFNC over NPPV as first-line treatment in patients with AHRF. During HFNC balancing, on an individual basis, the advantages and potential harmful effects of spontaneous breathing helps in identifying patients most likely to benefit from the treatment. Strict monitoring remains mandatory in order to identify, without delay, patients needing intubation and protective invasive ventilation.

Keywords: non-invasive ventilation, high-flow nasal cannula, spontaneous breathing, patient-self-inflicted lung injury, ventilator-induced lung injury, acute respiratory failure

Introduction

A vast variety of conditions, including pulmonary infection; inflammation; and exacerbation of chronic lung and heart disease may lead to acute hypoxemic respiratory failure (AHRF). AHRF and its sub-type (ARDS) characterized by lung injury; hypoxemia; altered respiratory mechanics; increased alveolar dead space; and vigorous respiratory drive.

High-flow nasal cannula (HFNC) together with conventional oxygen therapy (COT), continuous positive airway pressure (CPAP) and non-invasive positive pressure ventilation (NPPV), with helmet or face mask, comprise the types of non-invasive respiratory support for managing selected patients with AHRF. The aims of non-invasive respiratory support are to improve hypoxemia; to reduce work of breathing; to avoid intubation; to reduce mortality; and to buy time to effectively manage the precipitating factors.

Nevertheless, the management of AHRF is extremely challenging for ICU physicians. Although noninvasive support widely used in ICUs, it remains without solid evidence. Even in the most recent clinical practice guidelines [1] the European Respiratory Society (ERS) task force suggested (conditional recommendation) HFNC over COT and HFNC over NIV, based on moderate and very low certainty of evidence, respectively. Interestingly, it has long been shown that patients with AHRF, who have failed NPPV, exert a vigorous respiratory drive and have a poor prognosis [2]. Moreover, the dyssynchrony between the patient's high respiratory drive to breathe and the pressure support delivered by NPPV may lead to high tidal volumes and may aggravate the already injured lung [2, 3].

Thus, for the management of AHRF, it is of paramount importance:

a) To reduce patient's intense respiratory efforts in order to protect the injured lung [4];
b) To control patient's tidal volume to avoid further lung injury;
c) To balance the potential benefits of noninvasive respiratory support (i.e., maintenance of spontaneous breathing and avoidance of intubation) with the dangers of delayed intubation.

In particular, the benefits of HFNC are known to be both clinical (easy use; patient comfort; humidification; enhanced bronchial secretion clearance) and physiological (augmented air flow of up to 60 L/min meeting the inspiratory needs of the dyspnoeic patient with AHRF; achievement of stable FiO_2 as high as 100%; provision of low level of positive end-expiratory pressure (PEEP) facilitating alveolar recruitment; CO_2 wash-out of upper airway; improved ventilation and decreased work of breathing and decreased risk of self-inflicted lung injury (P-SILI).

The aim of this chapter is to discuss the benefits and potential harmful effects of spontaneous breathing; to present the main pathophysiological mechanisms by which the patient's inspiratory effort during HFNC could become injurious; and to address the potential clinical implications.

Physiological Aspects of Spontaneous Breathing

During the application of HFNC and other non-invasive respiratory support modalities (NPPV and CPAP) in patients with moderate-to-severe AHRF and ARDS, spontaneous breathing balances interesting advantages against ominous disadvantages, including further injury to the lung and diaphragm.

Benefits of Spontaneous Breathing during HFNC

HFNC is an open system permitting spontaneous breathing, which has long been introduced as an alternative modality of oxygen administration in non-intubated patients with AHRF. As such, the physiological functions related to airway protection (e.g., cough, clearance of secretions) preserved during HFNC therapy. Furthermore, by averting endotracheal intubation, complications related directly to intubation (e.g., laryngeal, and tracheal trauma) and to invasive mechanical ventilation (e.g., ventilation induced lung injury; ventilator associated pneumonia; sedation; neuromuscular blockade) are reduced. Finally, by keeping the patient alert and cooperative, delirium, discomfort and agitation also are greatly reduced.

The beneficial effects of spontaneous breathing also extended to the lung, diaphragm, and heart. Unassisted breathing increases the aeration of the dependent (dorsal) lung zones improving ventilation/perfusion matching and, thus, gas exchange. Moreover, intact inspiratory muscle tone promotes expansion of chest-wall and lungs at end expiration and in this way, it recruits previously closed lung zones and improves functional residual capacity [5, 6].

During spontaneous breathing, the active contraction of the diaphragm averts its disuse, dysfunction, and atrophy. Importantly, during inspiration, the dorsal portion of the diaphragm moves preferentially improving the ventilation of the dorsal lung zones, whereas during expiration, diaphragmatic activity might preserve lung volume and protect against lung collapse [7]. Finally, spontaneous breathing is associated with increased venous return and augmentation of cardiac output in pre-load dependent patients.

Potential Harmful Effects of Spontaneous Breathing during HFNC

The vicious circle deriving from hypoxemia, increased respiratory drive, abnormal respiratory mechanics, and inhomogeneous lung inflation, comprises the fundamental mechanism of the potential harmful effects during spontaneous breathing in patients suffering from ARDS. The causes of the dysregulated respiratory drive include hypoxemia and/or hypercapnia; metabolic acidosis; altered respiratory mechanics (decreased compliance, increased resistance); inflammation; fever; pain and agitation.

These factors result in increased inspiratory effort and consequently, in high tidal volumes, tachypnea and exaggerated transpulmonary swings, thereby positioning the already injured lung at increased risk of barotrauma, volutrauma and atelectrauma. The vigorous inspiratory effort together with the lung inhomogeneity and the pendelluft phenomenon comprise the key components of the mechanism recently introduced as P-SILI.

The intense inspiratory effort, as estimated by the deflection in the oesophageal pressure, exerts the following consequences. Firstly, it results in inflation of high tidal volume in lung regions with compromised aerated areas caused by edema, inflammation, and atelectasis. Therefore, high regional transpulmonary pressure and over-distension are generated mostly at the beginning of inspiration, which shifts fresh gas from the non-dependent (ventral) to dependent (dorsal) lung zones. This phenomenon is termed "pendelluft" and creates a high dorsal tidal volume and cyclic opening/closing of the dependent regions (which are collapsed during expiration) further worsening the lung injury (atelectrauma) [5].

Secondly, strong inspiratory effort creates negative deflections in pleural pressure which in turn transiently decrease the alveolar and lung interstitial pressures, ending up in increased transmural pulmonary capillary pressure and increased alveolar edema. Thirdly, intense inspiratory effort promotes inhomogeneity in the regional strength of the diaphragm resulting in inflammation, sarcolemma rupture and injury [5].

Although the concept of P-SILI is based on physiological and experimental data and some clinical observations, no clinical trial, to date, has demonstrated its relevance. It is also important to note that P-SILI is supposed to occur when a large inspiratory effort imposed on a previously injured lung. In an experimental study, Yoshida et al., demonstrated that intense inspiratory effort and severe prior lung injury worsened lung damage [8]. Conversely, in animals with mild lung injury, high inspiratory effort improved lung injury. Furthermore, data from endurance-trained healthy individuals showed that extreme transpulmonary pressure swings ($\leq$60 cmH_2O) and tidal volume >3L did not result in lung damage [6]. Thus, the mechanisms of P-SILI need to be elucidated. Until then, we should keep in mind that not all AHRF and ARDS patients have the same risks of P-SILI. A patient's inspiratory effort is proportional to the severity of his condition.

Additionally, patients with the most severe forms of AHRF (PaO_2/FiO_2 < 150-200 mmHg) are more susceptible to P-SILI. Finally, it is important to note that clinical studies have demonstrated that persistent high inspiratory effort is strongly associated with non-invasive respiratory support failure and the need for intubation.

Strategies to Make Spontaneous Breathing Less Injurious during High-Flow Oxygen

General Measures

As a first step, all the factors leading to dysregulated respiratory drive (e.g., hypoxemia and/or hypercapnia; metabolic acidosis; fever; pain and agitation) should be corrected.

Pharmacologic Agents

Theoretically, pharmacologic agents could be administrated to reduce respiratory drive. Although propofol and benzodiazepines are the only agents that have shown to reduce respiratory effort, they should be used only in highly selected patients because of their serious side-effects. Opioids are known to reduce respiratory frequency and dyspnea, but they have irregular effects on tidal volumes and respiratory effort. Importantly, opioids can control respiratory drive when it derives from pain. The major side effect of them is apnea and this is the reason, why a close monitoring is needed. Although dexmedetomidine (a selective alpha-2 agonist), in contrast to propofol and benzodiazepines, provides analgesia and anxiolysis, without respiratory depression, it does not reduce respiratory effort.

Application of PEEP

It has been demonstrated that HFNC generates a low and variable level of PEEP (2-7 cmH_2O) depending on the flow of gases delivered; on whether the mouth is open or closed; on the patient's sex and size. In contrast to HFNC, during therapy with NPPV, PEEP can be adjusted to higher values.

Careful application of PEEP may be useful in achieving lung and diaphragm protection because:

a) In recruitable lungs, PEEP decreases the amount of atelectatic units and, thus, reduces the vertical inspiratory gradient of transpulmonary pressure swings between non-dependent and dependent lung regions facilitating a more homogeneous distribution of ventilation [9];

b) PEEP reduces inspiratory effort without affecting respiratory drive (neuro-muscular uncoupling) by reducing the diaphragmatic curvature and improving the force-length relationship caused by the increase in end-expiratory lung volume [9]. Interestingly, this neuro-muscular uncoupling reduces inspiratory effort and tidal volume rendering spontaneous breathing less deleterious;

c) PEEP reduces air-hunger during low tidal volume ventilation resulting in improvement of patient-ventilator interactions;

d) PEEP may reduce excessive expiratory braking of the diaphragm, thereby averting injurious eccentric diaphragmatic load.

It has been reported that the diaphragm is an important regulator of expiration, acting as a brake during expiration to prevent lung collapse [7]. It is important to keep in mind that the above-mentioned advantages of PEEP should always be balanced with the risk of lung overdistension.

Application of Non-Invasive Respiratory Support Modalities

The discussion about the use of either mask-NPPV or helmet-NPPV as techniques to make intense respiratory efforts less deleterious for lung injury is not in the scope of this chapter.

High-Flow Nasal Cannula

High-flow oxygen is provided through a wide-bore nasal cannula by an air/oxygen blender which is directly connected to a flow meter; by a gas-compressed based ventilator; or by a turbine connected to an oxygen flow meter and a heated humidifier.

The most important and interdependent mechanisms by which HFNC could improve outcomes in AHRF are:

a) *Heating and humidification of inhaled gas.* HFNC delivers totally conditioned gas at a temperature of 37°C and an absolute humidity of 44 cmH_2O/L (relative humidity of 100%).

b) *High inspiratory flow.* HFNC provides predetermined high flow rates exceeding the value of 60 L/min, and fractions of inspired O_2 (FiO_2) up to 100% that can be independently adjusted. These advantages fill unmet needs for increased inspiratory flow in patients with dyspnea, acute hypoxemic respiratory failure and ARDS.
c) *Decreased entrainment of inspired room air and provision of* higher and more stable FiO_2 than the conventional oxygen delivery devices.
d) *Augmented wash-out of upper airways* that results in decreased anatomic dead space, decreased minute ventilation requirement, and reduced inspiratory effort and work of breathing.
e) *Generation of low and variable level of PEEP (2-7cmH$_2$O)*, which is proportional to HFNC flow rate.

In a small physiological study, with a cross-over design, Mauri et al., compared HFNC (flow of 40 L/min) to COT (12 L/min) in patients with AHRF by using an oesophageal catheter and electrical impedance tomography [10]. They found that HFNC improved oxygenation; effectively reduced respiratory effort and respiratory rate; and reduced minute ventilation to obtain a normal $PaCO_2$. They also reported that HFNC increased end-expiratory lung volume (EELV) in both dependent and non-dependent lung zones; improved dynamic compliance; and increased transpulmonary pressures while reducing transpulmonary driving pressures. This reduction in transpulmonary driving pressure suggested that HFNC might reduce stress inside the already injured lung.

More recently, in a prospective randomized cross-over study, Artaud-Macari et al., [11] by using the same technique (electrical impedance tomography) in patients with AHRF, compared, for the first time, the alveolar recruitment between HFNC and NPPV (pressure support level set to obtain an expiratory tidal volume of 6-9 mL/kg body weight (primary end-point)). They also compared lung volumes, respiratory and hemodynamic parameters; dyspnea, and patients' comfort between HFNC and NPPV, relative to face mask (secondary endpoint). They demonstrated increased EELV (PEEP effect) during HFNC and NPPV suggesting a potential benefit in alveolar recruitment with both techniques related to a face mask. More specifically, NPPV increased EELV, relative to COT, both in global lung and dependent and non-dependent lung zones, including the consolidation areas. Moreover, HFNC relative to COT with a face mask significantly increased EELV in global lung as well as in dependent lung areas, but without any harmful effects on global or regional tidal volume.

Interestingly, NPPV also increased tidal volume compared to HFNC and a face mask, while HFNC did not increase tidal volume relative to a face mask. The latter findings suggested that NPPV may contribute to lung overdistention with its deleterious effect in AHRF patients. Regarding oxygenation, NPPV achieved better SpO_2/FiO_2 indices compared to HFNC, whereas no significant difference in the dyspnea score was found between NPPV, HFNC and COT.

In their large multicenter, randomised, open-label, controlled trial, Frat et al., compared HFNO (50 L/min) vs COT vs intermittent sessions of face-NPPV in carefully selected patients with de novo AHRF (pneumonia in 75% of the patients) [12]. The primary endpoint (intubation rate) was not significantly different among the groups (HFNO 37% vs COT 47% vs NPPV 50% $p = 0.18$). However, in a post hoc adjusted analysis, the authors found that HFNO significantly reduced the intubation rate in patients with $PaO_2/FiO_2 \leq 200$ mmHg. Moreover, in the entire cohort HFNO increased ventilator-free days and reduced 90-day mortality with better comfort and less dyspnea. Surprisingly, NPPV patients had a worse 90-day mortality than HFNO patients, which was not easily explained. The authors speculated a higher risk of ventilator-induced lung injury, while tidal volume on NPPV exceeded 9 mL/kg of predicted body weight.

Nevertheless, it remains debatable whether the clinical outcome in this study was partly driven by P-SILI. It is known that HFNO can clear anatomical dead space from exhaled air and decrease rebreathing in a dose-dependent manner, making ventilation more efficient. This effect results in decreasing minute ventilation requirements and reducing inspiratory effort and labour of breathing. Many authors have suggested this as one of the major pathophysiological mechanisms that improve respiratory support, increase oxygenation, and reduce arterial and tissue CO_2. On a theoretical basis, HFNC could thus limit the risks of P-SILI compared to NPPV.

More recently, Grieco et al., [13] compared HFNC (flow of 50 L/min) with helmet-NPPV (pressure support ventilation10-15 cmH_2O and PEEP of 10-12 cmH_2O) in 15 patients with hypoxemia ($PaO_2/FiO_2 < 200$ mmHg) in randomized cross-over order. They found that the helmet-NPPV as compared with HFNC improved oxygenation and reduced dyspnea; inspiratory effort and simplified pressure-time product with similar transpulmonary pressure swings, PCO_2 and comfort. Interestingly, their findings were more pronounced in patients with vigorous baseline respiratory effort and more severe hypoxemia ($PaO_2/FiO_2 < 150$ mmHg).

In another multicenter, randomized controlled trial, the same group of investigators randomized 110 patients with COVID-19 and moderate-to-severe AHRF to either helmet-NPPV or HFNC [14]. They reported that there was no significant difference in the number of days free of respiratory support within 28 days (primary endpoint). Moreover, among 9 prespecified secondary outcomes, 7 showed no significant differences between the two groups. Treatment with the helmet-NPPV was associated with a significantly lower rate of endotracheal intubation and increased invasive ventilation-free days within 28 days. The authors underlined that further research is warranted to determine effects on other outcomes, including the need for endotracheal intubation. This study might also indicate that during NPPV, potential mechanisms of P-SILI are consistently associated with clinical outcomes.

The most recent ERS clinical practice guidelines suggested HFNC over COT and HFNC over NPPV in adults with AHRF based on moderate and low certainty of evidence, respectively [1]. They also suggested HFNC over COT during breaks of NPPV in patients for whom NPPV is chosen. Obviously, more evidence is needed a) to identify patients at high risk of deterioration and therefore more likely benefit from HFNC; and b) to evaluate the impact of HFNC versus NPPV in patients at different levels of risk of induced lung injury; different levels of PaO_2/FiO_2 severity; as well as in COVID-19 and other viral illnesses.

Monitoring Spontaneous Breathing during HFNC

Close monitoring is mandatory in non-intubated hypoxemic patients with ARF who managed with HFNC and NPPV. The early identification of patients at risk of HFNC failure is of paramount importance to avoid delayed intubation and poor outcomes. Vigorous inspiratory effort and high tidal volumes are known to be the major determinants for potential lung damage and a worse prognosis.

It is well known that monitoring and analysing waveforms of airway pressure, flow and tidal volume at the bedside are feasible and effective during invasive mechanical ventilation and NPPV. Conversely, it is extremely difficult, not to say almost impossible, to obtain these indices during HFNC.

The inspiratory swings in oesophageal pressure (Pes), as an estimation of pleural pressure, may provide a reliable assessment of respiratory effort even in non-intubated subjects undergoing HFNC and NPPV. Although precise values of respiratory effort, which is associated with high risk of non-invasive support failure, have not yet been defined, a ΔPes threshold of 15 cmH_2O has been proposed by some experts as a reasonable index.

Nevertheless, careful assessment of clinical data (dyspnea; hemodynamic and neurological status; recruitment of accessory respiratory muscles) and simpler modalities could be used at the bedside of moderately-to-severely hypoxemic patients during HFNC.

Continuous monitoring of oxygenation by pulse oximetry (SpO_2) is warranted during HFNC. However, it is important to note that pulse oximetry: a) is less reliable in critically ill patients compared to healthy individuals; b) is less accurate, as opposed to SaO_2, at low oxygen saturations; and c) is affected by the temperature-induced and the CO_2-induced shift in the oxygen dissociation curve.

Conversely, arterial blood gas analysis provides an accurate, albeit intermittent, estimation of gas exchange and oxygenation index (PaO_2/FiO_2). A PaO_2/FiO_2 ratio below 150-200 mmHg before treatment and/or a worsening trend of this that is associated with HFNC failure.

As respiratory rate is one of the vital signs, and a simple parameter to measure in everyday practice, it remains the most used surrogate of respiratory drive. It has been shown that severe lung injury is associated with intense inspiratory effort determining P-SILI and, thus, predicting the need of intubation in spontaneously breathing patients with AHRF. Nonetheless, in these patients, the respiratory rate reported to be a predictor of intubation under standard oxygen, but not under HFNC or non-invasive ventilation [15].

The ROX index, defined as the ratio of SpO_2/FiO_2 over respiratory rate, expresses the severity of hypoxemia combined with a surrogate of respiratory drive. The ROX index may predict the risk of HFNC failure and, thus, of intubation in AHRF patients. An index less than 2.85, less than 3.47, and less than 3.85 at 2, 6, and 12 hours respectively after HFNC initiation, are predictors of HFNC failure [16].

Conclusion

Current conditional guidelines suggest HFNC over COT and NPPV as first-line treatment in hypoxemic patients with PaO_2/FiO_2 >200 mmHg. During HFNC in patients with AHRF and ARDS, balancing the advantages against the disadvantages of spontaneous breathing is of paramount importance. Benefits of spontaneous breathing during HFNC include preservation of functions related to upper airway protection; avoidance of endotracheal intubation and its potential harmful effects; and protective lung and diaphragm ventilation.

Potential harmful effects of spontaneous breathing triggered by vigorous inspiratory effort include pendelluft phenomenon, P-SILI, deterioration of volutrauma, atelectrauma, negative pressure pulmonary edema, and diaphragmatic dysfunction. Close monitoring, especially among hypoxemic patients with a $PaO_2/FiO_2 < 200$ mmHg, is mandatory, taking into consideration clinical information; respiratory rate; pulse oximetry; arterial blood gases; and the ROX index. Follow the oesophageal pressure swings, whenever it is feasible, and keep $\Delta Pes < 15 cmH_2O$.

References

[1] Oczkowski S., Begüm Ergan, Lieuwe Bos, Michelle Chatwin, Miguel Ferrer, Cesare Gregoretti, Leo Heunks, Jean-Pierre Frat, Federico Longhini, Stefano Nava, Paolo Navalesi, Aylin Ozsancak Uğurlu, Lara Pisani, Teresa Renda, Arnaud W Thille, João Carlos Winck, Wolfram Windisch, Thomy Tonia, Jeanette Boyd, Giovanni Sotgiu, Raffaele Scala. ERS Clinical Practice Guidelines: High-flow nasal cannula in acute respiratory failure. *Eur Respir J,* 2021. Oct 28;2101574. doi: https://doi.org/10.1183/13993003.01574-2021.

[2] Carteaux G., Teresa Millán-Guilarte, Nicolas De Prost, Keyvan Razazi, Shariq Abid, Arnaud W Thille, Frédérique Schortgen, Laurent Brochard, Christian Brun-Buisson, Armand Mekontso Dessap. Failure of non-invasive ventilation for de novo acute hypoxemic respiratory failure: role of tidal volume. *Crit Care Med.* 2016. 44:282–290.

[3] Brochard L., Slutsky A., Pesenti A. (2017). Mechanical ventilation to minimize progression of lung injury in acute respiratory failure. *Am J Respir Crit Care Med,* 195:438–442.

[4] Yoshida T., Torsani V., Gomes S., De Santis R. R., Beraldo M. A., Costa E. L., Tucci M. R., Zin W. A., Kavanagh B. P., Amato M. B. Spontaneous effort causes occult pendelluft during mechanical ventilation. *Am J Respir Crit Care Med.* 2013. 188:1420–1427.

[5] Luca Grieco D., Salvatore Maurizio Maggiore, Oriol Roca, Elena Spinelli, Bhakti K. Patel, Arnaud W. Thille, Carmen Sílvia V. Barbas, Marina Garcia de Acilu, Salvatore Lucio Cutuli, Filippo Bongiovanni, Marcelo Amato, Jean-Pierre Frat, Tommaso Mauri, John P. Kress, Jordi Mancebo, Massimo Antonelli. Non-invasive ventilatory support and high-flow nasal oxygen as first-line treatment of acute hypoxemic respiratory failure and ARDS. *Intensive Care Med,* (2021). 47:851–866. https://doi.org/10.1007/s00134-021-06459-2.

[6] Carteaux G., Mélodie Parfait, Margot Combet, Anne-Fleur Haudebourg, Samuel Tuffet, Armand Mekontso Dessap. Patient-Self Inflicted Lung Injury: A Practical Review. *J Clin Med,* (2021). 10;2738. https://doi.org/10.3390/jcm10122738.

[7] Pellegrini M., Göran Hedenstierna, Agneta Roneus, Monica Segelsjö, Anders Larsson, Gaetano Perchiazzi.The Diaphragm Acts as a Brake during Expiration to Prevent Lung Collapse. *Am J Respir Crit Care Med.* 2017. 195:1608–1616.

[8] Yoshida T., Uchiyama A., Matsuura N., Mashimo T., Fujino Y. The Comparison of Spontaneous Breathing and Muscle Paralysis in Two Different Severities of Experimental Lung Injury. *Crit. Care Med.* 2013.41:536–545.

[9] Morais C. C. A., Yukiko Koyama, Takeshi Yoshida, Glauco M. Plens, Susimeire Gomes, Cristhiano A. S. Lima, Ozires P. S. Ramos, Sérgio M. Pereira, Naomasa Kawaguchi, Hirofumi Yamamoto, Akinori Uchiyama, João B. Borges, Marcos F. Vidal Melo, Mauro R. Tucci, Marcelo B. P. Amato, Brian P. Kavanagh, Eduardo L. V. Costa, Yuji Fujino. High Positive End-Expiratory Pressure Renders Spontaneous Effort Non-injurious. *Am J Respir Crit Care Med,* (2018). 197: 1285–1296.

[10] Mauri T., Turrini C., Eronia N., Grasselli G., Volta C. A., Bellani G., Pesenti A. Physiologic effects of high-flow nasal cannula in acute hypoxemic respiratory failure. *Am J Respir Crit Care Med*, (2017). 195: 1207–1215.

[11] Artaud-Macari E., Michael Bubenheim, Gurvan Le Bouar, Dorothée Carpentier, Steven Grangé, Déborah Boyer, Gaëtan Béduneau, Benoit Misset, Antoine Cuvelier, Fabienne Tamion, Christophe Girault. High-flow oxygen therapy versus non-invasive ventilation: a randomised physiological crossover study of alveolar recruitment in acute respiratory failure. *ERS Open Res*. (2021) 7(4):00373-2021.

[12] Frat J. P., Thille A. W., Mercat A., Girault C., Ragot S., Perbet S., Prat G., Boulain T., Morawiec E., Cottereau A., Devaquet J., Nseir S., Razazi K., Mira J. P., Argaud L., Chakarian J. C., Ricard J. D., Wittebole X., Chevalier S., Herbland A., Fartoukh M., Constantin J. M., Tonnelier J. M., Pierrot M., Mathonnet A., Béduneau G., Delétage-Métreau C., Richard J. C., Brochard L., Robert R.; FLORALI Study Group; REVA Network. High-flow oxygen through nasal cannula in acute hypoxemic respiratory failure. *N Engl J Med.* (2015). 372:2185–2196.

[13] Grieco D. L., Menga L. S., Raggi V., Bongiovanni F., Anzellotti G. M., Tanzarella E. S., Bocci M. G., Mercurio G., Dell'Anna A. M., Eleuteri D., Bello G., Maviglia R., Conti G., Maggiore S. M., Antonelli M. Physiological comparison of high-flow nasal cannula and helmet noninvasive ventilation in acute hypoxemic respiratory failure. *Am J Respir Crit Care Med*, (2020). 201:303–312.

[14] Grieco D. L., Menga L. S., Cesarano M., Spadaro S., Bitondo M. M., Berardi C., Rosà T., Bongiovanni F., Maggiore S. M., Antonelli M.; COVID-ICU Gemelli Study Group. Effect of helmet non-invasive ventilation vs high-flow nasal oxygen on days free of respiratory support in patients with COVID-19 and moderate to severe hypoxemic respiratory failure: the HENIVOT randomized clinical trial. *JAMA*. 2021. 325: 1731–1743.

[15] Frat J. P., Ragot S., Coudroy R., Constantin J. M., Girault C., Prat G., Boulain T., Demoule A., Ricard J. D., Razazi K., Lascarrou J. B., Devaquet J., Mira J. P., Argaud L., Chakarian J. C., Fartoukh M., Nseir S., Mercat A., Brochard L., Robert R., Thille A. W.; REVA network. Predictors of intubation in patients with acute hypoxemic respiratory failure treated with a non-invasive oxygenation strategy. *Crit Care Med.*2018. 46:208–215.

[16] Roca O., Berta Caralt, Jonathan Messika, Manuel Samper, Benjamin Sztrymf, Gonzalo Hernández, Marina García-de-Acilu, Jean-Pierre Frat, Joan R Masclans, Jean-Damien Ricard. An Index Combining Respiratory Rate and Oxygenation to Predict Outcome of Nasal High-Flow Therapy. *Am J Respir Crit Care Med.* (2019). 199: 1368–1376.

Chapter 10

Ventilatory Mode Approaches

Mario Agreda Fernández*, MD
Medical Health Science, Emergency Department,
Ramón y Cajal University Hospital, Madrid, Spain

Abstract

Non-invasive mechanical ventilation (NIV) is a non-invasive technique that confers provision of ventilatory support through the patient's upper airway using a mask or similar device. The goal of NIV is the improvement of gas exchange and clinical outcome in several types of acute respiratory failure. This technique has proven to be successful in correcting hypoventilation in selected conditions such as chronic obstructive pulmonary disease (COPD) exacerbations, cardiogenic pulmonary edema, restrictive chest wall diseases or acute asthma.

Several randomized studies have demonstrated its benefits by mainly decreasing the need for endotracheal intubation and its associated complications as invasive procedure. Compared to invasive ventilation, NIV has also shown to reduce weaning time, decrease rates of nosocomial pneumonia, improve survival rates and reduce hospital length of stay. Its use has dramatically increased in the last decade.

Pressure support ventilation (PSV) is an assisted ventilatory mode of NIV where the ventilation is patient-triggered (by pressure, airflow, or both), pressure-limited, and flow cycled. In this modality, the airway pressure is maintained almost constant during the entire inspiration. The ventilator provides assistance when the patient makes a breathing effort, and then, when inspiratory flow reaches a certain threshold level, cycling to exhalation occurs.

* Corresponding Author's Email: agrefermd@gmail.com.

In: Ventilator Induced Lung Injury in Non-Invasive Ventilatory Support
Editor: Antonio M. Esquinas
ISBN: 979-8-88697-840-7

Keywords: non-invasive ventilation, asthma, acute respiratory failure, cardiogenic pulmonary edema, COPD exacerbation, nosocomial pneumonia, survival rate

Introduction

Positive-pressure ventilation (PPV) is a form of respiratory therapy that involves the delivery of air, or a mixture of oxygen combined with other gases by positive pressure into the lungs. PPV had its greatest initial boom at the 1950s to treat acute respiratory failure during the poliomyelitis outbreaks. PPV can be delivered in two forms: non-invasive pressure support ventilation (NIPSV), which is delivered through the patient's upper airway using a special face mask with a tight seal (air travels through anatomical airway), or invasive pressure support ventilation (IPSV), which involves the delivery of positive pressure to the lungs through an endotracheal tube or tracheostomy [1, 2].

Non-Invasive Pressure Support Ventilation: Ventilatory Modes

The use of NIPSV has markedly increased over the last two decades and has now become an integral tool in the management of both acute and chronic respiratory failure [3-5]. NIPSV is considered a supportive therapy that can be lifesaving if started properly. The major benefit of NIPSV is the avoidance of deep sedation for endotracheal intubation and the attendant risks of invasive mechanical ventilation such as nosocomial infections or ventilator-associated pneumonia. NIPSV has even become a more sophisticated technique and operator friendlier than IPSV.

NIPSV provides support spontaneously during the patients' inspiratory breathing effort, and then, when inspiratory flow reaches a certain threshold level, cycling to exhalation occurs. In this modality, the airway pressure is maintained almost constant during the entire inspiration. NIPSV has shown to be more effective than "continuous positive airway pressure" (CPAP) at unloading the respiratory muscles, improving cardiac and hemodynamic function [6]. In the NIPSV setting, the operator sets the percentage of flow assistance for the current volume. The amount of pressure provided and FiO_2 should be adjusted. The respiratory cycle can be limited by pressure or by time cycle.

This modality of ventilation requires two levels of pressure: expiratory positive airway pressure (EPAP) and inspiratory positive airway pressure (IPAP). The pressure support (PS), the real ventilatory support that the patient would obtain, is measured by the difference between them. The process takes place during both stages of the respiratory cycle. During the inspiration air flow decelerates to maintain the pressure support (PS) triggered by patient's effort. The result is a continuous positive pressure added to the spontaneous pressured triggered by the patents' effort during inspiration. During the expiration, the target is providing ventilatory support by a positive end-expiratory pressure (PEEP). The main indications of NIPSV are acute cardiogenic pulmonary edema (ACPE), acute heart failure (AHF), chronic obstructive pulmonary disease (COPD) exacerbations, hypercapnic respiratory failure and weaning from mechanical ventilation.

Ventilator Setting

NIPSV is usually started with inspiratory pressures of 8–12 cmH_2O and expiratory pressures of 4–5 cmH_2O. Patients´ collaboration is crucial and requires clear explanations from the attending team and the appropriate use of sedation if needed.

Once the patient is comfortable with the initiation of the ventilator support, the IPAP should be increased up to 15-20 cmH_2O and EPAP to 5-8 cmH_2O. The ventilator should detect when it needs to deliver the programmed IPAP or "inspiratory trigger." Current barometric ventilators use faster and more sensitive flow triggers (lower patient effort and shorter response time). The ventilator should also detect when to end the inspiratory phase (drop in the flow delivered) and allow the patient to initiate the expiration phase. This is called "expiratory trigger" or "expiratory cycling." This flow fall can be preset, either by a preset value in the ventilator software or by giving the programmer the possibility of modifying it according to the entity treated [7]. Figure 1.

A "target respiratory rate" should be programmed and it needs to be lower than the patients´ respiratory rate. The ventilator will detect when a period of bradypnea or apnea occurs. Visual evaluation of the patients´ breathing effort and breathing rhythm is another important mean to optimize patient ventilator synchrony.

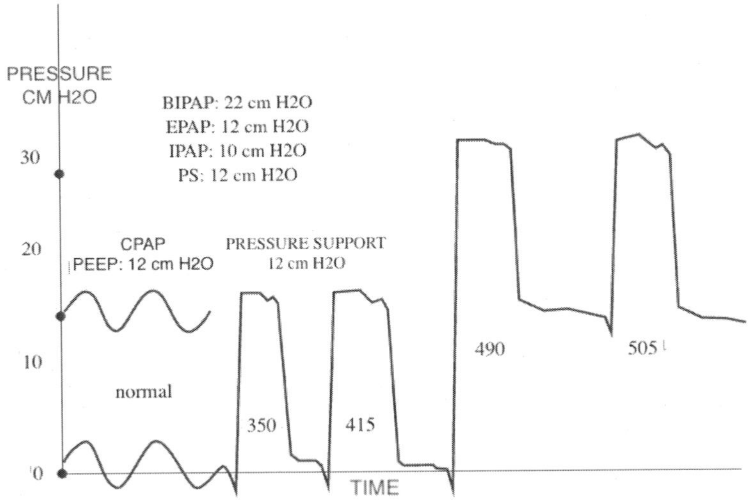

Figure 1. Pressure/time curves in spontaneous, continuous positive airway pressure (CPAP) and BiPAP, Pressure support (PS). Positive end expiratory pressure (PEEP), Inspiratory positive airway pressure (IPAP), expiratory positive airway pressure (EPAP).

This mode of ventilation has some disadvantages such as the need of expertise for ventilator setting in order to reduce over-assistance when the patient increases its inspiratory effort and the accessibility to an appropriate device. Besides, compared with invasive mechanical ventilation it can be poorly tolerated in an awake patient, ventilation may be less effective due to air leaks, and it should only be used for short periods. It has also some limitations such as the need for patient collaboration and contraindications (listed in Table 1).

Table 1. Contraindications to non-invasive ventilation

Need for emergent intubation (egg, cardiac or respiratory arrest, severe respiratory distress, unstable cardiac arrhythmia)
Non-respiratory organ failure that is acutely life-threatening
Severe encephalopathy (GCS < 10)
Severe upper gastrointestinal bleeding
Hemodynamic instability
Facial or neurological surgery, trauma or deformity
Significant airway obstruction (e.g., laryngeal mass or tracheal tumor)
Inability to cooperate, protect airway, or clear secretions (e.g., patients at high risk or aspiration)
Anticipated prolonged duration of mechanical ventilation (e.g., > 4-7 days)

GCS: Glasgow Coma Score.

Complications

Complications related to NIPSV are few (less than 5%), generally minor, and often related to the mask employed (e.g., local irritation or ulceration, air leaks, nasal dryness or congestion, gastric distension, and aspiration). The major concern is the risk of barotrauma, which is partially prevented by lung-protective ventilation and occurs less frequently than with invasive ventilation [8]. Potential risks and lung complications are summarized in Table 2.

Table 2. Lung complications associated with non-invasive mechanical ventilation

Mechanical complications
Barotrauma (volutrauma)
Pneumothorax
Pneumomediastinum
Biotrauma
Atelectrauma
Infectious complications
Aspiration pneumonia

Barotrauma

Administration of positive pressure by a mechanical ventilator has its own attendant problems. Patients receiving positive-pressure ventilation are subject to *barotrauma*: traumatic changes such as pneumothorax or pneumomediastinum occurring due to high alveolar pressures. Because alveolar overdistention with rupture is currently thought to be the cause of these complications, the term, *volutrauma*, has now taken over for *barotrauma*.

Concern has been raised that the excessive volumes and high levels of pressure provided to the alveoli may be injurious to alveolar structures. Considering lung injury in acute respiratory distress syndrome (ARDS), including pulmonary edema is often heterogeneously distributed being inspiratory gas preferentially dispersed to the healthy territories. The ventilator continues to deliver gas under positive pressure, and the gas enters the pleural space through the rupture. The pressure in the pleural space and thorax increases, and a *tension pneumothorax* can result, which critically diminishes venous return and cardiac output and causes rapid cardiovascular collapse.

Development of a *pneumothorax* could lead to catastrophic consequences if not detected and treated quickly. In such situations, we need to treat as soon as possible by decompressing the pleural space with a tube, catheter, or needle to allow resumption of venous return, and to permit expansion of the lung.

Biotrauma

The concept of *biotrauma* was proposed by Slutsky and colleagues [9] who showed that the high volume tidal (Vt) ventilation led to expression of inflammatory mediators and neutrophil recruitment as a biological answer of biophysical factors and showed this harm a part of multiple organ dysfunction. This puts the more normal alveoli at particular risk for overdistention. At the same time, more diseased alveoli are subject to collapse (atelectasis) during the expiratory phase of the respiratory cycle because of intra-alveolar fluid and/or a disrupted or insufficient surfactant layer. Alveoli that are open during inspiration but collapse during expiration are subject to abnormal shear stresses during the repetitive process of opening and closing, a complication termed *atelectrauma.*

Both alveolar overdistention and atelectrauma may be accompanied by microscopic injury to cells of the alveolar wall and to intercellular attachments, leading to disruption of the normal permeability barrier provided by alveolar epithelial and capillary endothelial cells. In addition, proinflammatory cytokines may be released, a phenomenon that has been called *biotrauma*, resulting in ongoing alveolar injury and systemic effects such as increasing the likelihood of developing multiorgan dysfunction syndrome.

In order to reduce this damage, Slutsky et al., proposed to maintain what they called a "permissive hypercapnia," based on the finest handling of pressure levels, it was the beginning of the lung protection strategy [9]. This strategy contributed to the reduction of morbidity and mortality of ventilated patients.

Aspiration Pneumonia

Aspiration pneumonia (AP) has been reported at least in 5% of patients treated with NIPSV. To minimize the rates of aspiration pneumonia is important an adequate management of secretions, with special attention to those patients with compromised upper airway function or with problems in clearing secretions. Nasogastric tube could be inserted if the patient has gastric distension, ileum or vomiting. Nasogastric tubes should not be routinely used because they interfere with mask fitting and promote air leaking.

Conclusion

Noninvasive mechanical ventilation (NIV) is a non-invasive technique that confers provision of ventilatory support through the patient's upper airway using a mask or similar device. Although The goal of NIV is the improvement of gas exchange and clinical outcome, its necessary to take into account the there are some complex pathophysiology mechanisms that could impact negatively in lung mechanic physiology such as barotrauma/ biotrauma and its appropriate an early monitoring and appropriate ventilatory setting.

References

[1] Mehta S, Hill N S (2001) Noninvasive ventilation. *Am. J. Respir. Crit. Care Med.* 163:540–577.

[2] Masip J. Non-invasive ventilation. *Heart Fail. Rev.* 2007;12(2):119-124. doi:10.1007/s10741-007-9012-7.

[3] Comellini V, Pacilli A M G, Nava S. Benefits of non-invasive ventilation in acute hypercapnic respiratory failure. *Respirology.* 2019 Apr;24(4):308-317. doi: 10.1111/resp.13469. Epub 2019 Jan 12. PMID: 30636373.

[4] Pisani L, Nava S. Noninvasive ventilation in acute hypercapnic respiratory failure. *Semin. Respir. Crit. Care Med.* 2014 Aug;35(4):501-6. doi: 10.1055/s-0034-1383864. Epub 2014 Aug 11. PMID: 25111646.

[5] Masip J, Peacock W F, Price S, Cullen L, Martin-Sanchez F J, Seferovic P, et al. Indications and practical approach to non-invasive ventilation in acute heart failure. *Eur. Heart J.* 2018;39(1):17-25. doi:10.1093/eurheartj/ehx580.

[6] Chadda K, Annane D, Hart N, Gajdos P, Raphael J C, Lofaso F (2002) Cardiac and respiratory effects of continuous positive airway pressure and non-invasive ventilation in acute cardiac pulmonary edema. *Crit. Care Med.* 30:2457–2461.

[7] Seyfi S, Amri P, Mouodi S. New modalities for non-invasive positive pressure ventilation: A review article. *Caspian J. Intern. Med.* 2019;10(1):1-6. doi:10.22088/cjim.10.1.1.

[8] Carron M, Gagliardi G, Michielan F, Freo U, Ori C (2007) Occurrence of pneumothorax during noninvasive positive pressure ventilation through a helmet. *J. Clin. Anesth.* 19:632–635.

[9] Curley G F, Laffey J G, Zhang H & Slutsky A S (2016). Biotrauma and Ventilator-Induced Lung Injury: Clinical Implications. *Chest*, *150*(5), 1109–1117. https://doi.org/10.1016/j.chest.2016.07.019.

Chapter 11

High Frequency Non-Invasive Ventilation

Deniz Heppekcan*, MD
Intensive Care Department,
Darica Farabi Training and Education Hospital, Kocaeli, Turkey

Abstract

High frequency non-invasive ventilation (HF-NIV) technique is a brand new approach that used in the implementation of the lung imaging procedures that require sustained apnea for the stabilization of the thoracic movements during the breathing. HF-NIV applied with the same principles as high frequency ventilation (HF-V), which is an invasive mechanical ventilation mode that provides oxygen delivery and carbon dioxide excretion, although there is no chest movement in anesthetized and invasively ventilated people. it is performed using a non-invasive interface and provides prolonged apnea in awake (non-sedated) patients.

The use of a high frequency ventilation technique with a non-invasive interface has been used not as a treatment modality for respiratory failure, but in PET/CT or MR imaging of the lung. The most important reason for using the HF-NIV technique in all these approaches is that it allows a safe and stabilized inspiration for the patient. Such an application would be of interest for several clinical applications, e.g., lung imaging and radiotherapy treatment on lung cancer. As a result, this system has been adapted in recent years for use in procedures requiring prolonged apnea, such as suppression of respiratory movement.

Keywords: high frequency non-invasive ventilation, respiratory stabilization, lung, lung imaging

---

* Corresponding Author's Email: denizheppekcan@yahoo.com.tr.

In: Ventilator Induced Lung Injury in Non-Invasive Ventilatory Support
Editor: Antonio M. Esquinas
ISBN: 979-8-88697-840-7

Introduction

Using HFV with a noninvasive interface (HF-NIV) to achieve prolonged apnea (absence of respiratory movements) is a new approach that has been explored in recent years for the lung imaging and radio-therapy procedures.

Although computed tomography (CT) is the first-choice modality for detailed chest imaging, the potential hazard of exposure to high doses of radiation remains a health concern. At this point, although the capabilities of magnetic resonance imaging (MRI) are tempting, it has suffered from its sensitivity to respiration and heart movement [1]. Combined PET/computed tomography (CT) is the most important imaging modality in the diagnosis, follow-up and treatment planning of malignancies [2]. Thoracic and abdominal mobility caused by respiratory movement make challenges in both quality of the PET/CT and MR imaging. To obtain high-resolution and appropriate MR imaging without respiratory artefacts, a technique that allows the acquisition when the lung is fully expanded at the end of inspiration is required. In addition, this technique, which provides a decrease in respiratory movements, can reduce the amount of normal lung parenchyma irradiated during radiotherapy of lung cancer.

HFV has previously been used in patients under general anesthesia to suppress thoracic and abdominal motions [3, 4]. However, a method that can be applied in awake (non-sedated) patients, can prevent respiratory artifacts and provide prolonged apnea on inspiration will be safer and more comfortable.

The need for a prolonged apnea period that provides thorax stabilization of at the end of the inspiration in order to suppress respiratory artifacts and allow for an accurate lung analysis has led researchers to study the method such as HF percussive ventilation and pulsative flow ventilation with a noninvasive interface. In several studies conducted in recent years, it has been shown that HF-NIV is applied in awake (non-sedated) and spontaneously breathing (non-intubated) patients and provides stabilization in thoracoabdominal movements during lung imaging and radiotherapy with prolonged apnea obtained during inspiration.

In the studies, the application of HFV using a noninvasive interface allowed a significant prolongation of apnea time in awake healthy subjects compared with spontaneous apnea, while preserving normal oxygen and carbon dioxide levels [1-4].

High-Frequency Percussive Ventilation (HFPV) or Pulsative-Flow Ventilation (PFV)

Péguret et al., firstly used the modified HFPV (or pulsatile flow ventilation TM) technique (Percussionaire; Idaho, USA) to achieve apnea-like respiratory motion stabilization at full inspiration for lung imaging and radiation therapy, and apnea lasting 8-16 minutes, which allows radiation therapy in non-intubated patients [5]. Based on the principle that the higher the respiratory frequency, the less the chest will move, the inspiratory time of was set to an infinite value and the expiration time to the minimum value during the chest stabilization period. Airway pressures were adjusted between 20 and 35 cm H_2O, percussion frequency was adjusted between 300 and 600 breaths/min depending on tolerance. This technique, which can suppress respiratory movement showed for the first time the applicability and tolerability of the high frequency percussive ventilation with a mouthpiece interface, allowing chest RT under prolonged apnea like breath hold.

Similarly, Prior et al., used pulsatile-flow ventilation with noninvasive technique, for the reduction of respiratory movement during PET/CT imaging. It was the first clinical evaluation for use of HF-NIV in this field [6]. The technique was developed to provide continuous apnea-like chest stabilization in conscious, non-intubated, spontaneously breathing patients. it was also suppressing low-frequency cycles to maintain adequate oxygen and carbon dioxide pressures without respiratory movement. In this study, PFV-induced apnea was shown to be clinically feasible for at least 8.5 minutes.

In another study, PFV with non-invasive technique was used to chest MRI and long-term stabilization of lung volumes with marked reduction in respiratory motion at full inspiration were demonstrated during MRI scans [7]. Experiences in the efficacy and safety evaluations of the using prolonged apnea supported by high frequency non-invasive ventilation technique in the fields of thoracic MRI, PET/CT and radiotherapy are increasing day by day [8-11].

Conclusion

High frequency non-invasive ventilation, which was developed to achieve apnea-like respiratory motion stabilization at full inspiration, apnea lasting 8-16 minutes can be achieved in non-intubated patients, which allows radiation therapy or medical imaging. In all patients administered HF-NIV, intrinsic respiratory movement was suppressed and the diaphragm was in the maximal inspiratory position, and oxygen saturation remained normal (95-100% under 100% fraction of inspired oxygen). HF-NIV also allowed for image quality improvements, especially for vascular and airway acuity of the whole chest. Many studies show that the technique was safe and well tolerated by all the study participants, with dryness of the upper airways being the main reported discomfort.

References

[1] Higano N S, Hahn A D, Tkach J A, Cao X, Walkup L L, Thomen R P, Merhar S L, Kingma P S, Fain S B, Woods J C. Retrospective respiratory self-gating and removal of bulk motion in pulmonary UTE MRI of neonates and adults. *Magn. Reson Med.* 2017;77:1284–1295.

[2] Pépin A, Daouk J, Bailly P, Hapdey S, Meyer ME. Management of respiratory motion in PET/computed tomography: the state of the art. *Nucl. Med. Commun.* 2014;35(2):113-122. doi:10.1097/MNM.0000000000000048.

[3] Denys A, Lachenal Y, Duran R, Chollet-Rivier M, Bize P. Use of high-frequency jet ventilation for percutaneous tumor ablation. *Cardiovasc. Intervent. Radiol.* 2014 Feb;37(1):140-6. doi: 10.1007/s00270-013-0620-4. Epub 2013 May 2. PMID: 23636246.

[4] Chung D Y, Tse D M, Boardman P, Gleeson F V, Little M W, Scott S H, Anderson EM. High-frequency jet ventilation under general anesthesia facilitates CT-guided lung tumor thermal ablation compared with normal respiration under conscious analgesic sedation. *J. Vasc. Interv. Radiol.* 2014 Sep;25(9):1463-9. doi: 10.1016/j.jvir.2014.02.026. Epub 2014 May 10. PMID: 24819833.

[5] Péguret N, Ozsahin M, Zeverino M, Belmondo B, Durham A D, Lovis A, Simons J, Long O, Duclos F, Prior J, Denys A, Beigelman C, Sozzi W J, Grant K, Gautier-Dechaud V, Peters S, Vienne M, Moeckli R, Bourhis J. Apnea-like suppression of respiratory motion: First evaluation in radiotherapy. *Radiother. Oncol.* 2016 Feb;118(2):220-6. doi: 10.1016/j.radonc.2015.10.011. PMID: 26979264.

[6] Prior J O, Péguret N, Pomoni A, Pappon M, Zeverino M, Belmondo B, Lovis A, Ozsahin M, Vienne M, Bourhis J. Reduction of Respiratory Motion During PET/CT by Pulsatile-Flow Ventilation: A First Clinical Evaluation. *J. Nucl. Med.* 2016 Mar;57(3):416-9. doi: 10.2967/jnumed.115.163386. Epub 2015 Dec 3. PMID: 26635339.

[7] Beigelman-Aubry C, Peguret N, Stuber M, Delacoste J, Belmondo B, Lovis A, Simons J, Long O, Grant K, Berchier G, Rohner C, Bonanno G, Coppo S, Schwitter J, Ozsahin M, Qanadli S, Meuli R, Bourhis J. Chest-MRI under pulsatile flow ventilation: A new promising technique. *PLoS One.* 2017 Jun 12;12(6):e0178807. doi: 10.1371/journal.pone.0178807. PMID: 28604833; PMCID: PMC5467845.

[8] Ogna A, Bernasconi M, Belmondo B, Long O, Simons J, Peguret N, Heinzer R, Nicod LP, Bourhis J, Lovis A. Prolonged Apnea Supported by High-Frequency Noninvasive Ventilation: A Pilot Study. *Am. J. Respir. Crit. Care Med.* 2017 Apr 1;195(7):958-960. doi: 10.1164/rccm.201608-1572LE. PMID: 28362201.

[9] Delacoste J, Dournes G, Dunet V, Ogna A, Noirez L, Simons J, Long O, Berchier G, Stuber M, Lovis A, Beigelman-Aubry C. Ultrashort echo time imaging of the lungs under high-frequency noninvasive ventilation: A new approach to lung imaging. J Magn Reson Imaging. 2019 Dec;50(6):1789-1797. doi: 10.1002/jmri.26808. Epub 2019 May 28. Erratum in: *J. Magn. Reson Imaging.* 2021 Feb;53(2):642. PMID: 31136048; PMCID: PMC6900075.

[10] Darçot E, Delacoste J, Dunet V, Dournes G, Rotzinger D, Bernasconi M, Vremaroiu P, Simons J, Long O, Rohner C, Ledoux JB, Stuber M, Lovis A, Beigelman-Aubry C. Lung MRI assessment with high-frequency noninvasive ventilation at 3 T. *Magn. Reson Imaging.* 2020 Dec;74:64-73. doi: 10.1016/j.mri.2020.09.006. Epub 2020 Sep 6. PMID: 32898653.

[11] Audag N, Van Ooteghem G, Liistro G, Salini A, Geets X, Reychler G. Intrapulmonary percussive ventilation leading to 20-minutes breath-hold potentially useful for radiation treatments. *Radiother. Oncol.* 2019 Dec;141:292-295. doi: 10.1016/j.radonc.2019.09.024. Epub 2019 Oct 25. PMID: 31668897.

Chapter 12

A Summary of Animal Studies and Clinical Implications

Alejandro Úbeda Iglesias[1,*], MD, PhD and Irene Fernández Burgos[2], MD

[1] Intensive Care Unit, Hospital Punta de Europa, Algeciras, Spain
[2] Intensive Care Unit, Regional University Hospital of Málaga, Málaga, Spain

Abstract

Ventilator-induced lung injury (VILI) is a serious acute injury to the lung tissue that can develop during mechanical ventilation (MV). Due to the mechanical strain of ventilation, damage can occur in the bronchiolar and alveolar epithelium resulting in a cascade of events that may be fatal to the patients [1]. The practice of positive-pressure ventilation has undergone a significant change. Most important in the past decade is the preference to use noninvasive ventilation (NIV).

Although NIV prevents the complications of intubation, it has potential to cause harm, especially in patients with *de novo* respiratory failure [2]. Patients requiring NIV are often critically ill, which limits the possibility of obtaining patient samples, making VILI research challenging. *In vitro* models are very important for VILI research, but the complexity of the cellular interactions in multi-organ animals, necessitates *in vivo* studies. However, the settings and duration of ventilation used to create VILI in mice vary greatly, causing uncertainty in interpretation and comparison of results [1].

* Corresponding Author's Email: alubeda@gmail.com.

In: Ventilator Induced Lung Injury in Non-Invasive Ventilatory Support
Editor: Antonio M. Esquinas
ISBN: 979-8-88697-840-7

Keywords: non-invasive ventilation, lung injury, lung deflation, effort-induced lung injury, lung stress

Introduction

During normal inspiration, air flows into the lungs due to negative pressure generated in the thorax by expanding the lungs via contraction of the diaphragm and intercostal muscles. During NIV, the opposite occurs, air is thrust into the lungs with the use of positive pressure, which can lead to damage of the lung epithelium due to mechanical strain, named VILI.

Consequently, NIV can exacerbate respiratory failure in already diseased lung tissue, or even be the primary cause of it through VILI in healthy lungs. Table 1 summarizes the mechanisms of VILI during positive pressure ventilation in patients with *de novo* respiratory failure.

Table 1. Mechanism of VILI during PPV in patients with *de novo* respiratory failure

Mechanism of VILI	PPV parameter	Management during NIV
Volutrauma	High tidal volume	If tidal volume continues to be high, then abort NIV and intubate early
Biotrauma	High tidal volume and low PEEP	If tidal volume continues to be high, then abort NIV and intubate early
Atelectrauma	High respiratory rate and low PEEP	Increase PEEP

PPV: positive pressure ventilation.

Volutrauma

Volutrauma represents VILI caused as lung units are overdistended with increased transpulmonary pressure. Animal studies have demonstrated that high tidal volumes (or high lung volumes), rather than high airway pressure *per se*, cause lung injury. Large tidal volumes (TV) are not always required for alveolar overdistension. When there is heterogeneous consolidation or atelectasis, a disproportionate volume from each breath is delivered to the open alveoli. This can cause regional alveolar overdistension and VILI despite delivery of conventional TV that are based upon body weight. A similar process is at play when lung compliance is reduced such as severe fibrosis or during single lung ventilation when a tidal breath is distributed to only one lung [3].

Atelectrauma

Atelectrauma is proposed as an additional possible form of VILI attributable to MV. Tidal ventilation at low airway pressure (starting from below and finishing above the lower inflection point determined from an inspiratory volume/pressure curve) can augment lung injury by cyclic opening and closing of airway and pulmonary units. A theoretical model was constructed which suggest that the forces effectively acting on the lung parenchyma can be much higher than those applied to the airway [4].

Biotrauma

Biotrauma is characterized by ventilator-induced release of inflammatory mediators from cells within the injured lung. Alveolar overdistension and atelectrauma have been shown in animals to result in an increase in inflammatory mediators (neutrophils, macrophages, and likely alveolar epithelial cells) including tumor necrosis factor (TNF-alpha), interleukin IL-6, IL-8 and matrix metalloproteinase-9 [5]. There is also evidence that injurious ventilatory strategies may lead to the subsequent development of pulmonary fibrosis (in animals) [6], although the precise mechanisms are unclear. However, many of the strategies that target inflammation in acute respiratory distress syndrome (ARDS) and VILI have not been successful [7].

Pathophysiology of VILI

The Role of End-Inspiratory Stress/Strain

VILI can only occur in ventilated regions. Inflammatory lung edema resembling clinical ARDS consistently has been induced in animals with healthy lungs using extremely high TV (usually 20–40 mL/kg body weight) and airway pressure (as high as 35–45 cmH2O). The safety of a particular TV or airway pressure cannot be judged without considering the size of the ventilated lung and the mechanical properties of the chest wall. This becomes even more important during lung disease. The total lung capacity (TLC) of a normal 70-kg adult male is usually considered to be approximately 7.5 L, with a resting lung volume (functional residual capacity [FRC]) of approximately 2.5 L.

According to these values, the upper limit for physiologic strain is normally reached when the lung volume is increased two-fold relative to end expiration. In other words, maximal strain should be equal to 2, considering the strain as the ratio between the volume of gas inflated (7.5–2.5 L) and FRC (2.5 L). At this level of strain, the collagen fibers of the lung fibrous skeleton are likely to be completely unfolded. Any attempt to further expand the lung will probably result in tissue rupture. If we consider the quasi-linear part of the lung volume/transpulmonary pressure curve, the relationship between the two variables is described by the following equation:

$$\text{Stress} = K * \text{strain}$$

where K is the lung-specific elastance (13 cmH_2O in either healthy or acutely injured lungs) [8].

Accordingly, if strain is equal to 2, transpulmonary pressure (TP) will be approximately 26 cmH_2O. The airway pressure corresponding to these values of TP strictly depends on the relationship between lung and chest wall elastances. We may expect lung injury to occur whenever the upper limit of physiologic strain is exceeded. Strain would then be equal to 2, TP would be approximately 26 cmH_2O, and airway pressure would be approximately 37 cm H_2O [8].

If we cautiously move this threshold down to the point where the relationship between strain and stress becomes curvilinear (75% of TLC), then TV of at least 3 L (45 mL/kg) would be required to induce VILI. The corresponding strain would then be equal to 1.2 and transpulmonary pressure would be 14 cm H_2O. The corresponding airway pressure would be approximately 20 cm H_2O. A TV of this order of magnitude (45 mL/kg) has been shown to produce VILI in mice [9].

Gattinoni et al., [4] proposed a model in which end-expiratory lung volume and the TLC represent the two extremes in which VILI may occur. When we consider values, the maximal physiologic strain should be approximately 2. We may then conclude that a strain more than 2 cannot be reached without rupturing the lung fibers. They observed that in adult surgical patients with healthy lungs, FRC measured by helium dilution is on average 1.7 L, which is a value lower than predicted. Accordingly, any given TV will correspond to different strain levels depending on whether FRC is estimated or directly measured. Height, age, body position, sedation and paralysis, and changes in abdominal pressure may all significantly impact on the lung volume at rest.

Because the maximal physiologic strain occurs at TLC, it would seem logical to define the strain as the ratio between end inspiratory lung volume and TL. In this case, the maximal physiologic strain would be 1 (end-inspiratory lung volume TLC). Unfortunately, estimation and measurement of TLC can be as tricky as those of FRC. Therefore, although the concept of strain either referenced to FRC or TLC is based on a strong physiologic premise, the variability of gas volume for any given amount of lung tissue can be so large that its definition and clinical utility may be not straightforward. Another possible approach to the definition and computation of strain could be to refer it to the amount of ventilated lung tissue.

For any given TV, strain will be obviously greater when delivered into an ARDS lung than into a healthy one, simply because the lung open to ventilation is smaller during acute lung injury; this concept has been described as "baby lung." The relevant issue here is whether the baby lung is more fragile *per se* and susceptible to VILI. The anatomical changes that occur during acute lung injury apparently do not alter the mechanical characteristics of the regions open to ventilation. Because the extracellular matrix is, at the same time, the main determinant of lung mechanics and bears most of the stress/strain attributable to mechanical ventilation, it seems that the available evidence is not sufficient to conclude that the baby lung is more prone to VILI compared to the healthy lung.

The Role of End-Expiratory Stress/Strain

Mead et al., [10] suggested that any lung damage attributable to mechanical ventilation is amplified whenever lung units collapse at end expiration and reopen at the next inspiration. They provided a theoretical model that can be oversimplified: the forces acting on a collapsed lung structure are far greater than those acting on an already expanded region because the surface bearing the force is diminished. The alveolar surface expands according to the power of two-thirds of any volume increase.

Even if we separately considered the TV and PEEP phenomena, in reality they are likely to be strictly interwoven. The amount of tissue that remains open at end expiration or that may undergo intra-tidal opening and closing depends on the TV previously delivered and the corresponding inspiratory pressure [11]. The potential danger effect of high TV may then be not only attributable to high TV *per se* (end-inspiratory phenomenon) but also may depend on the increased amount of tissue undergoing cyclic opening and closing (end-expiratory phenomenon).

According to the model proposed by Mead [10], the major amplification of distorting forces occurs at the interface between open and constantly closed pulmonary units. If recruitment occurs during inflation, then the alveolar surface bearing the applied force will augment and the local amplification of force will decrease accordingly.

Research on VILI

Clinical research on VILI in patients is challenging due to the high-risk nature of invasive diagnostic procedures in patients with serious respiratory failure. Access to patient lung samples is therefore limited, effectively restricting research to either healthy tissue or end-point samples; emphasizing the need for alternative methodologies such as *in vitro* research, or *in vivo* animal models.

Mice have been extensively used to study VILI. However, there is no standardized model for establishing VILI in mice in the literature and important parameters in published papers vary considerably. These key parameters include choice of TV, time of ventilation, breaths per minute, use of protective ventilation strategies such as PEEP, choice of anesthetic drugs, type of animal used, and whether it is appropriate to base the ventilation on pressure or tidal volume generated by the mechanical ventilator. Such variation creates difficulties in reproducing an equivalent, robust model, as well as interpretation and comparison of results [1].

Alternative Animal Experimentation

In vitro models of VILI are few and physiologically limited. The lung is a complex organ and contains several epithelial, interstitial, and immune cell types arranged in a wide variety of tissues within the organ, which is extremely difficult to recapitulate *in vitro*. Cell models usually do not adequately represent the mechanical forces that lung tissues and cells *in vivo* are subjected to. Joelsson et al., conducted a novel *in vitro* system to mimic VILI in lung epithelial cells cultured in air–liquid interface conditions, using the cyclical pressure air–liquid interface device (CPAD) [12]. Employing the CPAD, they were able to mimic important events in VILI by inducing barrier damage in bronchial and alveolar epithelial cell layers. They showed that azithromycin treatment protected the epithelial layer against mechanical strain by maintaining the actin structures of the cytoskeleton, changing lipid metabolism, and attenuating inflammatory responses [12]. *In vitro* systems are useful to gain an initial indication of relevant mechanisms, but they lack the complex epithelium, stroma and the microvasculature interactions. Therefore, translation of results from *in vitro* studies to clinical usefulness requires testing in *in vivo* models.

On the other hand, the importance of the inflammatory response in the prognosis of VILI has been studied. In a mouse model of VILI, mechanical ventilation with high tidal volume promoted the accumulation of lung neutrophils, leading to increased IL-17 levels in the lung. Depletion of neutrophils decreases the production IL-17 in mice and inhibition of IL-17 significantly reduced lung injury and inflammatory response [13]. Moreover, a study showed that other interleukin, IL-10, may regulate the inflammatory response in the lung tissue, improve lung tissue oxygenation, and inhibit oxidative stress, therefore reducing VILI in rats [14].

The fact that *in vitro* lung models are gaining popularity among researchers that are increasingly avoiding animal testing, and the difficulty in gaining human samples for lung research make this pressure system a very relevant tool for use in lung and drug testing research.

Finally, novel bioinformatics analysis has focused on investigating the differential expression gene in mice with VILI. Dysregulation of genes related to immune responses has been positively correlated with the development of VILI. Moreover, Chen et al., [15] performed an analysis based on genomic datasets and found that VILI was mainly related to inflammatory injury, cytokines, and immune cell infiltration; IL-1**β**, suppressor of cytokine signaling 3 (SOCS3) and matrix metalloproteinase-9 (MMP-9) might be biomarkers of VILI.

Conclusion

Consider that:

- MV can harm the lung.
- VILI is an acute injury to the lung which appears during MV due to the mechanical strain of ventilation.
- VILI may occur in ventilated regions and can be divided in volutrauma, atelectrauma and biotrauma.
- *In vitro* lung models are gaining popularity.
- Early biomarkers of VILI are needed; genomics may have the solution.

References

[1] Joelsson J P, Ingthorsson S, Kricker J, Gudjonsson T, Karason S. Ventilator-induced lung-injury in mouse models: Is there a trap? *Lab. Anim. Res*. 2021;37:30.

[2] Katira B. Ventilator-Induced Lung Injury: Classic and Novel Concepts. *Respiratory Care* June 2019;64:629-37.

[3] Pietro Caironi, Massimo Cressoni, Davide Chiumello, Marco Ranieri, Michael Quintel, Sebastiano G Russo, Rodrigo Cornejo, Guillermo Bugedo, Eleonora Carlesso, Riccarda Russo, Luisa Caspani, Luciano Gattinoni. Lung opening and closing during ventilation of acute respiratory distress syndrome. *Am. J. Respir. Crit. Care Med.* 2010; 181:578.

[4] Gattinoni L, Protti A, Caironi P, Carlesso E. Ventilator-induced lung injury: The anatomical and physiological framework. *Crit. Care Med.* 2010;38:S539-48.

[5] Gattinoni L, Carlesso E, Cadringher P, Valenza F, Vagginelli F, Chiumello D. Physical and biological triggers of ventilatorinduced lung injury and its prevention. *Eur. Respir. J. Suppl*. 2003; 47:15s–25s.

[6] Pietro Caironi, Massimo Cressoni, Davide Chiumello, Marco Ranieri, Michael Quintel, Sebastiano G Russo, Rodrigo Cornejo, Guillermo Bugedo, Eleonora Carlesso, Riccarda Russo, Luisa Caspani, Luciano Gattinoni. Lung recruitment in patients with the acute respiratory distress syndrome. *N. Engl. J. Med*. 2006; 354: 1775–86.

[7] Miller A J, Spence J R. *In vitro* models to study human lung development, disease and homeostasis. *Physiology* (Bethesda) 2017;32:246–60.

[8] Davide Chiumello, Eleonora Carlesso, Paolo Cadringher, Pietro Caironi, Franco Valenza, Federico Polli, Federica Tallarini, Paola Cozzi, Massimo Cressoni, Angelo Colombo, John J Marini, Luciano Gattinoni. Lung stress and strain during mechanical ventilation for acute respiratory distress syn- drome. *Am. J. Respir. Crit. Care Med.* 2008; 178:346 –55.

[9] Caironi P, Ichinose F, Liu R, Jones R C, Bloch K D, Zapol W M.. 5-Lipoxygenase Deficiency Prevents Respiratory Failure during Ventilator-induced Lung Injury. *Am. J. Respir. Crit. Care Med.* 2005;172:334-43.

[10] Mead J, Takishima T, Leith D. Stress distribution in lungs: A model of pulmonary elasticity. *J. Appl. Physiol.* 1970; 28:596-608.

[11] Tommaso Mauri, Takeshi Yoshida, Giacomo Bellani, Ewan C Goligher, Guillaume Carteaux, Nuttapol Rittayamai, Francesco Mojoli, Davide Chiumello, Lise Piquilloud, Salvatore Grasso, Amal Jubran, Franco Laghi, Sheldon Magder, Antonio Pesenti, Stephen Loring, Luciano Gattinoni, Daniel Talmor, Lluis Blanch, Marcelo Amato, Lu Chen, Laurent Brochard, Jordi Mancebo, PLeUral pressure working Group (PLUG—Acute Respiratory Failure section of the European Society of Intensive Care Medicine). Esophageal and transpulmonary pressure in the clinical setting: meaning, usefulness and perspectives. *Intensive Care Med.* 2016;42:1360-73.

[12] Jon P Joelsson, Iwona T Myszor, Ari J Arason, Saevar Ingthorsson, Paulina Cherek, Gabriel S Windels, Kristjan Leosson, Gudmundur H Gudmundsson, Thorarinn Gudjonsson, Sigurbergur Karason Innovative *in vitro* method to study ventilator induced lung injury. *Altex.* 2019;36:634-42.

[13] Xiaoting Liao, Weikang Zhang, Huijun Dai, Ren Jing, Mengling Ye, Wanyun Ge, Shenglin Pei, Linghui Pan. Neutrophil-derived IL-17 promotes ventilator-induced lung injury via p38 MAPK/MCP-1 pathway activation. *Front. Immunol.* 2021;12: 768813.

[14] Chen J, Lin J, Luo H, Li M. Effects of human interleukin-10 on ventilator-associated lung injury in rats. *Inflammation* 2019;42:538-47.

[15] Chen S, Zhang Y, Zhan Q. Bioinformatics analysis of ventilator-induced lung injury genome microarray based on gene expression omnibus database and key gene verification. Zhonghua Wei Zhong Bing Ji Jiu Yi Xue 2022;34:41-7.

Chapter 13

Pathophysiology, Treatment and Prevention

Lucía Hinojosa Díaz*, **MD**
Emergency Department, Río Hortega Hospital, Valladolid, Spain

Abstract

Non-invasive mechanical ventilation can result both acute lung injury and worsen pre-existing lung injury as well as multiorgan failure due to the release of inflammatory mediators into the systemic circulation. This is called ventilator-induced lung injury (VILI).

Four mechanisms of VILI have been demonstrated: barotrauma, volutrauma, atelectrauma and biotrauma. Diagnosis is basically clinical with features like acute respiratory distress syndrome (ARDS), knowing that in this case it is caused by mechanical ventilation.

Over the years, through studies comparing different ventilator parameters, ventilation strategies have been established that are effective in protecting lung to prevent VILI. Preventing overdistention of functional lung units by using small tidal volumes (6 ml/kg predicted body weight) and maintaining a plateau pressure of ≤ 30 cm H_20 can minimize damage.

Keywords: ventilator-induced lung injury, non-invasive mechanical ventilation, acute respiratory distress syndrome, acute lung injury, preventing ventilation

* Corresponding Author's Email: luciahinojosa14@gmail.com.

In: Ventilator Induced Lung Injury in Non-Invasive Ventilatory Support
Editor: Antonio M. Esquinas
ISBN: 979-8-88697-840-7

Introduction

Non-invasive mechanical ventilation is a supportive treatment in patients with respiratory failure, but it presents complications or perpetuates lung injury and multiorgan failure due to the release of inflammatory mediators into the systemic circulation. This injury occurs both in healthy lungs and in pre-existing lung injury, being more usual and serious in patients with pre-existing lung injury [1].

At present, the optimal purpose of ventilation is to keep the patient alive, ensuring good arterial oxygen pressure (PaO2) or arterial oxyhaemoglobin saturation (SaO2) and minimize adverse consequence of mechanical ventilation.

First, it is necessary to clarify a series of concepts:

1) *Ventilator-induced lung injury (VILI)*: it is lung injury that is caused by or exacerbated by mechanical ventilation. It is similar to acute respiratory distress syndrome (ARDS). International Consensus Conferences in Intensive Care Medicine described it in 1998. Mainly is seen in patients with ARDS but VALI has also been shown to occurs in patients ventilated for other reasons.
2) *Ventilator-associated lung injury (VALI)*: it is lung injury produced during mechanical ventilation and whose cause cannot be proven. VILI would be that VALI produced by the ventilator itself.
3) *Self-induced lung injury (SILI)*: it is lung injury that is caused by an excessive tidal volume due to the spontaneous efforts of the patient.

Pathophysiology

Four mechanisms defined in the production of VILI [1]: barotrauma, volutrauma, atelectrauma and biotrauma. All of this causes alveolar injury that results in high alveolar permeability, lung edema, alveolar hemorrhage, and loss of pulmonary surfactant, alveolar collapse and multiorgan failure [2-3].

Barotrauma

It is conceptually as lung injury caused by excessive airway pressure (high transpulmonary pressure) while volutrauma is lung injury caused by alveolar overdistention. However, these two mechanisms have proven their relationship over the years.

In 1974, Webb and Tierney published a study that showed lung injuries caused by excessive airway pressure in rats ventilated with different pressure levels and with/without positive end-expiratory pressure (PEEP). It observed that the injury was caused by lung overdistention, so we could talk more about volume damage than pressure damage. Furthermore, the absence of injury demonstrated when only the volume limited, while when the pressure limited, the same thing did not occur. These phenomena have also demonstrated in other animals such as rabbits or sheep and in humans through different pressure and volume strategies.

Atelectrauma

Defined as lung injury caused consequence of the cyclical process of opening (expansion in inspiration) and closing (collapse in expiration) of alveoli that gives rise to atelectatic alveoli. These atelectatic alveoli causes shear forces that result in injury to neighboring non-atelectatic alveoli and nearby airways. Surfactant dysfunction and edematous lung contribute to regional atelectrauma. This phenomenon is induced by low circulating volume in relation to insufficient PEEP. There are studies that show that adequate early PEEP prevents lung injuries in patients with mechanical ventilation.

Biotrauma

Biotrauama refers to the process that, through previous mechanisms, produces not only in the alveolar space but also in the systemic circulation a release of inflammatory mediators. In this way, extrapulmonary organ system injury is produced and thus it is also demonstrated that in patients who have died due to VILI, multiorgan failure occurs, renal failure (also cardiovascular, hepatic failure). Cytokines are released that function as inflammatory mediators, inducing the release of other mediators, recruiting neutrophils, and increasing vascular permeability which allows the translocation of these substances to the blood territory. The translocation of bacteria to the systemic circulation producing bacteremia has also demonstrated. In summary is additional lung and extrapulmonary organ injury by proinjurious inflammatory response to mechanical lung injury.

Other ventilator parameters have also been shown to contribute to VILI, although in a less significant way. In a certain way, a high respiratory rate can worsen lung injury an increase in pulmonary edema and perivascular hemorrhage. The use of decelerating flow instead of constant flow with decreased lung distention has also been studied.

All these mechanisms give rise to more serious and evident injury in previously damaged or immature lungs compared to healthy lungs.

Diagnosis

Table 1. Alternative causes of respiratory failure

ARDS	HSCT
Sepsis	Pancreatitis
Pneumonia (aspiration or infectious pneumonia: bacterial, viral, fungal, and parasitic)	Transfusion related acute lung injury and massive transfusion
Severe trauma	Drugs
Burns and smoke inhalation	Thoracic or other major surgery
Embolism	Intra-abdominal distension
Lobar collapse	Pleural effusion
Acute coronary syndrome	

Diagnosis of VILI is based on clinical features; these are similar to ARDS, along with the exclusion of alternative causes of respiratory failure [4, 5]. We consider some key aspects for diagnosis:

1) *Clinical features:* VILI appears in patients as a need for a higher oxygen requirement to maintain the same oxygen pressure (pO2) or arterial oxyhemoglobin saturation (SatO2). Patients present dyspnea and on physical examination we will be able to observe tachypnea and/or tachycardia, diaphoresis, and diffuse crackles. In severe cases patients may be present acute confusion or respiratory distress. Always keep in mind that it occurs secondary to ventilation.
2) *Diagnostic test:* chest radiography will request showing new or worsening bilateral interstitial or alveolar infiltrates. On computed tomography (CT) of the chest these injuries will be more evident as areas of heterogeneous consolidation, areas of atelectasis, as well as pulmonary overdistention.

In addition, laboratory test (including lipase, cardiac enzymes, coagulation), arterial blood gas analysis, electrocardiogram may also request to exclude alternative causes.

3) *Alternative causes:* ARDS, new pulmonary infection and lung edema are the most common etiologies to be excluded. Other etiologies to rule out described in Table 1.

Treatment and Prevention

Patients with VALI will be treated in the same way as those with ARDS and those without. It must be keep in mind that one of the greatest challenges in patients receiving mechanical ventilation and that do not present ARDS is the balance between a protective ventilation strategy but one that does not worsen the underlying pathology [6, 7]. Therefore, we have to use scales that allow us to identify patients who are more susceptible to presenting with acute lung injury, although it has not been shown that the use of these scales should guide either treatment or prevention. Different management alternatives will be explained below:

Lung-protective ventilation: it is the essential initial measure before starting ventilation based on the use of low tidal volume, low plateau pressure and use of adequate PEEP. An arterial oxygen pressure of 55 to 80 mmHg or an oxygen saturation of 88 to 95% supported as a goal. In this way, it will be advisable to prescribe a tidal volume of 6 ml/kg of ideal weight and maintain a plateau pressure ≤ 30 cm H_20. This will have a significant impact on patient mortality as well as decrease in pulmonary hyperinflation. To avoid atelectrauma, we would adjust PEEP value to the fraction of inspired oxygen (FiO_2). There are studies also give importance to driving pressure (Driving pressure = plateau pressure – PEEP) as a key data to predict mortality, even more accurate if accurate if it is also related to respiratory rate, studies are still lacking to determine the true importance of these values. Regarding respiratory rate, it recommended to avoid the high frequency ventilation strategy (combination of respiratory rates > 60 breaths/minute with tidal volume less than anatomical dead space). Table 2. FiO_2 / PEEP combinations

Table 2. FiO_2 / PEEP combinations

FiO2	0.3	0.4	0.5	0.6	0.7	0.8	0.9	1.0
PEEP	5	5 to 8	8 to 10	10	10 to 14	14	14 to 18	18 to 24

Prone position: It refers to the administration of mechanical ventilation in prone position. It has been shown to be effective in patients with severe ARDS. Prone position is a strategy to improve oxygenation when traditional modes of ventilation fail. The benefit of prone ventilation is improved gas exchange due to improved ventral-dorsal transpulmonary pressure gradient, decreased dorsal pulmonary compression and improved pulmonary perfusion. It is not considered a ventilation mode properly.

Extracorporeal membrane oxygenation (ECMO): it is not considered as a first line to prevent VILI. Its efficacy is based on the improvement of gas exchange, also through the extracorporeal elimination of CO_2.

Conclusion

Ventilator-induced lung injury (VILI) defined as acute lung injury that occurs during mechanical ventilation. It is more common in patients with acute respiratory distress syndrome (ARDS), although it can also occur in patients who are receiving mechanical ventilation for other reasons than ARDS, even in patients with previously healthy lungs [8].

Four pathophysiological mechanisms causing VALI described such as: barotrauma, volutrauma, atelectrauma and biotrauma. All of this causes alveolar injury that results in high alveolar permeability, lung edema, alveolar hemorrhage, and loss of pulmonary surfactant, alveolar collapse and multiorgan failure [9, 10].

VALI is a clinical diagnosis with the clinical presentation of ARDS but in this case knowing that it is due to the use of mechanical ventilation. It is also necessary to exclude other diagnoses such as new pulmonary infection or pulmonary edema.

Prevention of VALI may decrease multiorgan failure and mortality. In treatment, it is important to use preventive ventilation strategies with proven efficacy, such as limiting tidal volume to 6 ml/kg of ideal weight or plateau pressure $\leq$ 30 cm H_2O, in addition to adjusting positive end-expiratory pressure (PEEP) according to FiO_2 [11, 12].

References

[1] Parker, James C., Lucrecia A. Hernandez, and Keith J. Peevy. "Mechanisms Of Ventilator-Induced Lung Injury." *Critical Care Medicine* 21, no. 1 (1993): 131-143.

[2] Webb H. H., Tierney D. F. Experimental pulmonary edema due to intermittent positive pressure ventilation with high inflation pressures. Protection by positive end-expiratory pressure. *Am. Rev. Respir. Dis.* 1974; 110: 556-565.

[3] John E., Ermacilla R., Golden J. Effects of intermittent positive pressure ventilation on lungs of normal rabbits. *Br. J. Exp. Pathol.* 1980; 61: 315-323.

[4] "International Consensus Conferences in Intensive Care Medicine: Ventilator-Associated Lung Injury In ARDS." *American Journal of Respiratory and Critical Care Medicine* 160, no. 6 (1999): 2118-2124.

[5] Gordo Vidal, F., C. Delgado Arnaiz, and E. Calvo Herranz. "Lesión Pulmonar Inducida Por La Ventilación Mecánica [*Mechanical Ventilation Induced Lung Injury*]." *Medicina Intensiva* 31, no. 1 (2007): 18-26. doi:10.1016/s0210-5691(07) 74765-4.

[6] Gattinoni, Luciano, John J. Marini, Francesca Collino, Giorgia Maiolo, Francesca Rapetti, Tommaso Tonetti, Francesco Vasques, and Michael Quintel. "The Future of Mechanical Ventilation: Lessons from The Present and The Past." *Critical Care* 21, no. 1 (2017).

[7] Donoso F., Alejandro, and Pablo Cruces R. "Daño Pulmonar Inducido Por Ventilación Mecánica Y Estrategia Ventilatoria Convencional Protectora [*Lung Damage Induced By Mechanical Ventilation And Protective Conventional Ventilatory Strategy*]." *Revista Chilena de Pediatría* 78, no. 3 (2007).

[8] Beitler, Jeremy R., Atul Malhotra, and B. Taylor Thompson. "Ventilator-Induced Lung Injury." *Clinics In Chest Medicine* 37, no. 4 (2016): 633-646.

[9] Rana, Sameer, Milie M. Tolentino, Rolf D. Hubmayr, Peter C. Gay, and Ognjen Gajic. "Risk factors for failure of non-invasive ventilation in patients with acute lung injury." *Chest* 128, no. 4 (2005): 226S.

[10] "Ventilation with Lower Tidal Volumes as Compared with Traditional Tidal Volumes for Acute Lung Injury and The Acute Respiratory Distress Syndrome." *New England Journal of Medicine* 342, no. 18 (2000): 1301-1308. "UpToDate." Uptodate.Com,2022.

[11] https://www.uptodate.com/contents/ventilator-induced-lung-injury?search=da%C3%B1o%20pulmonar%20inducido%20por%20ventilacion&source=search_result&selectedTitle=6~150&usage_type=default&display_rank=6.

[12] Verbrugge, S. J. C., V. Šorm, A. van 't Veen, D. Gommers, B. Lachmann, and J. W. Mouton. "Lung Overinflation Without Positive End-Expiratory Pressure Promotes Bacteremia After Experimental Klebsiella Pneumoniae Inoculation." *Intensive Care Medicine* 24, no. 2 (1998): 172-177.

Chapter 14

Non-Invasive Negative Pressure Ventilation and Prevention of Lung Injuries

Mohammad Sallam[1], MD
Nikhil Patankar[2], MD
and Omar Alibrahim[3,*], MD

[1] Boston Children's Hospital, Harvard Medical School, Department of Pediatrics, Boston, Massachussets, USA
[2] Beacon Children's Hospital, Beacon Health System. South Bend, Indiana, USA
[3] Duke University Medical Center, Duke Children's Hospital, Department of Pediatrics. Division of Pediatric Critical Care Medicine, Durham, North Carolina, USA

Abstract

The use of non-invasive ventilation (NIV) has increased in the past two decades for different indications in both pediatric and adult populations. Non-invasive positive pressure ventilation (NIPPV) is the most commonly used type of NIV. NIPPV, however, is not without risks. Ventilator-induced lung injury (VILI) can be seen in patients supported with NIPPV. This risk is in part caused by the "radical departure" from the normal breathing physiology during NIPPV utilization. Negative pressure ventilation (NPV) is another less commonly used type of NIV.

Current data suggests the efficacy of NPV and its favorable effects on both lung kinetics and hemodynamics. In this chapter, we summarize the main physiologic concepts of normal breathing, NIPPV, NPV, the factors associated with VILI, and NPV, the supporting literature, and the clinical considerations.

---

* Corresponding Author's Email: Omar.alibrahim@duke.edu.

In: Ventilator Induced Lung Injury in Non-Invasive Ventilatory Support
Editor: Antonio M. Esquinas
ISBN: 979-8-88697-840-7

Keywords: non-invasive ventilation, negative pressure ventilation, ventilator-induced lung injury, positive pressure ventilation, acute respiratory failure

Introduction

Since it showed efficacy and superiority to the iron lung during the poliomyelitis pandemic in the late 1950s [1], positive pressure ventilation has gained more value in the management of acute respiratory failure. Recent epidemiologic data suggests increasing utilization of both invasive [2] and non-invasive [3] positive pressure ventilation.

Non-invasive Positive Pressure Ventilation (NIPPV) use has been increasing in both pediatric and adult [4] patients with variable rates around the world [5]. It has been used for many clinical indications and pathologies (Table 1).

Table 1. The common acute clinical indications of NIPPV

Pediatric	Adults
- Parenchymal lung disease (pneumonia, atelectasis, bronchiolitis) - Lower airway disease (asthma) - Upper airway obstruction (croup, post extubation stridor) - Facilitation of weaning of mechanical ventilation - Avoiding intubation in patients at high risk for intubation (immunocompromised patients).	- Parenchymal lung disease (pneumonia, atelectasis) - Chronic Obstructive Pulmonary Disease (COPD) exacerbation - Lower airway disease (asthma) - Cardiogenic pulmonary edema - Facilitation of weaning of mechanical ventilation - Avoiding intubation in patients at high risk with intubation (immunocompromised patients)

Despite its "non-invasive" nature, NIPPV is not without risks [6, 7]. Concerns about NIPPV include the following:

- Facial and nasal pressure ulcers related to facemask or nasal mask application.
- Gastric distension with aspiration risk.
- Risk of loss of lung recruitment with suctioning and secretion clearance.
- Risk of delayed intubation and higher mortality after failure of NIPPV.

- Positive pressure related- lung injury (barotrauma, volutrauma).

Physiology of Positive Pressure Ventilation

While invasive and non-invasive positive pressure ventilation utilize different equipment, they both assist ventilation by the same physiological concept; the delivery of pressurized gas to the terminal airway [8-10].

Two physiologic concepts are essential to understand positive pressure ventilation as well as the differences between the physiologic basics of positive pressure, negative pressure and natural breathing:

First: The lung inflation pressure, also known as the transpulmonary pressure (Ptp) which can be mathematically represented by the following equation:

$$Ptp = Palv - Ppl$$

where Palv is the intra-alveolar pressure and Ppl is the intrapleural pressure.

The difference between the alveolar and the pleural pressure has to be positive for the alveoli to overcome their tendency to collapse. During normal inspiration, the respiratory muscles contraction causes the chest wall to be pulled outwards resulting in negative intrapleural pressure. This leads to the airflow inwards to the lungs, leading to alveolar distension causing positive transpulmonary pressure that favors alveolar inflation. Negative pressure ventilation utilizes the same physiologic concept, causing more negative intrapleural pressure and subsequently, more positive transpulmonary pressure causing lung recruitment. Positive pressure ventilation, on the other hand, inflates the alveoli by "pushing pressure" into the airway increasing Palv and Ppl and therefore, reverses the physiologic pattern of breathing.

Second: The gradient pressure (aka: driving pressure) that causes air movement into the alveoli. This gradient can be described by the following equation:

$$\text{Driving Pressure} = Pao - Palv$$

where Pao is the pressure at the airway opening (nose or mouth in natural airway and NIPPV, the end of the endotracheal tube, or the tracheostomy tube in invasive mechanical ventilation).

During natural breathing and negative pressure ventilation, the Palv drops as a result of respiratory muscle contraction leading to a pressure gradient that favors air entry into the alveoli. In positive pressure ventilation, on the other hand, the Pao is increased which creates a pressure gradient that moves air into the alveoli.

Table 2 describes the physiologic effects of positive pressure, negative pressure, and natural breathing on the lung-inflation pressure (transpulmonary pressure) and the driving pressure.

Table 2. Physiologic changes caused by positive and negative pressure ventilation and a comparison with natural breathing

Factor	Natural Breathing	Positive Pressure Ventilation	Negative Pressure Ventilation
Ppl	Negative	Variable. No patient effort: Positive Patient effort: Negative (due to triggering)	Negative
Ptp (Palv-Ppl)	Maintained by the negative Ppl	Maintained by increasing Palv	Maintained by increasing the "negativity of Ppl"
Pao	Atmospheric	Positive	Atmospheric
Driving Pressure (Pao-Palv)	Gradient caused by negative Palv	Gradient caused by increasing Pao	Gradient increased by more negative Palv

Ventilator Induced Lung Injury (VILI)

"Respirator lung" was one of the first terms used to describe the lung damage observed in patients after post-mechanical ventilation in 1967 [11]. Currently, the term ventilator induced lung injury (VILI) is used to describe the sequalae of positive pressure mechanical ventilation on normal and injured lungs. Which, at cellular level, is characterized by cellular infiltrates, increased vascular permeability, and pulmonary edema [12].

Physiology

Several factors play a role in the development of ventilator associated lung injury:

1) *Mechanical factors*: Including the non-physiologic high airway pressure, the overdistension and the cyclic collapse/distension of the alveoli during mechanical ventilation. These factors lead to three distinctive subtypes of mechanical injury:
   a. *Barotrauma*: Injury attributed to high airway pressure; specifically, the peak inspiratory pressure.
   b. *Volutrauma*: Injury attributed to alveolar overdistension.
   c. *Atelectotrauma*: Injury attributed to cyclic distension/collapse of the alveoli.
2) *Biological factors*: These include cellular reactions that occur secondary to the mechanical effect; mainly the overdistension and cyclic distension that leads to the activation of ion channels and protein mediated reactions in the alveolar epithelium and vascular endothelial cells leading to increased permeability, inflammatory cellular recruitment, and release of cytokines [13] .

Which Causes More Harm: The Pressure or the Volume?

One of the very first experimental studies that aimed to explore the potential harmful effect of high peak pressure on the animal lungs found that higher peak pressures with lower positive end expiratory pressure (PEEP) caused more harmful effects compared to lower peak pressure and higher PEEP [14]. This harmful effect of pressure and volume on ventilated lungs was further clarified by Dreyfuss et al. That study showed that only animal lungs exposed to high tidal volume developed lung injury when compared to animals exposed to the same peak pressure with lung expansion being restricted by thoracoabdominal strapping. This led to the conclusion that lung overdistension with higher tidal volume is more critical than high peak pressure as a causal factor of VILI [15].

Regional lung overdistension is important to be kept in mind as a key mechanism of VILI when ventilating sick lungs even when the overall tidal volume is not high. Limiting the inflation pressure should, therefore, be a target during positive pressure ventilation to minimize lung overdistension and its associated lung injury [16].

Could NIPPV be Harmful?

As discussed, overdistension is likely to be the most critical causal factor in VILI. Distension pressure can be described by the equation:

$$Ptp = Palv\text{-}Ppl$$

where pressure alv is the intra-alveolar pressure and Pp in the intrapleural pressure.

While the alveolar pressure might be higher in patients receiving invasive ventilation (due to upper airway resistance); NIPPV is not without overdistension risks. During NIPPV in distressed patients, the patients' effort creates more negative intrapleural pressure (Ppl) leading to even higher Ptp and lung distension pressure [16].

NPV Physiology

During spontaneous breathing, tidal volume is generated in the alveoli by creating a pressure gradient between the alveoli and the atmosphere leading to a pressure gradient that favors air entry into the alveoli. Spontaneous ventilation has numerous beneficial effects on the cardio-respiratory system, including maintaining diaphragmatic muscle mass and strength, improving ventilation-perfusion matching, thereby improving gas exchange, and maintaining systemic venous return. Studies have also shown that patient who breathe spontaneously need lesser sedation and thereby experience lesser sedation related side effects [[17]7]. By improving venous return, right ventricular (RV) end-diastolic volume and eventually RV stroke volume may increase [18].

NPV devices (i.e., RTX ventilator) work by exposing the surface of the chest wall to sub-atmospheric (negative) pressures resulting in recruitment of the alveoli and expansion of the lungs. The negative pressure can be maintained at a constant level throughout the respiratory cycle resulting in continuous negative extra thoracic pressure (CNEP), or the inspiratory and expiratory phases can be fully controlled with biphasic cuirass ventilation (BCV) by modifying the negativity of the air pressure (control mode).

This pressure causes lung expansion and draws atmospheric air into the lungs and the alveoli to promote gas exchange. In spontaneous ventilation, exhalation is passive. However, a negative pressure ventilator can generate positive pressure to compress the thorax, and this leads to an active exhalation, which further augments ventilation especially in a sick lung [19].

NPV Devices

The initial device used for delivering negative pressure ventilation was the "iron lung" or the "tank ventilator" in the era of poliomyelitis which encompassed the entire body except the head with an airtight seal around the neck. The device also had portholes through which patient access and monitoring was made possible. The tight seal around the neck increased risk of jugular vein obstruction and risk of hypothermia due to constant air flow within the tank. There have been several modifications to this device in the form of latex seal without pressure all around the neck and control of ambient air temperature to prevent hypothermia [19].

Pneumo-wrap or the "pulmo-wrap" was another device in the form of an airtight jacket or a poncho that seals around the neck, arms, and thighs with straps at the wrists and ankles that ensure airtightness. The poncho came in different sizes when connected to the ventilator can work in controlled and assisted modes [19].

The most recent device that is currently used to deliver NPV is via the chest cuirass (loosely translated from French word cuirasses which means a chest armor). The cuirass is a shell made of transparent plastic material and straps around the patient's anterior chest. An airtight seal across the patient's chest is achieved by tightening the fabric straps that can be velcroid together. Many sizes of the plastic shell are available to accommodate newborns to full grown adults. The cuirasses are available in 4 adult and 7 pediatric sizes. Once fitted and placed on the patient, the cuirass is then connected to the Hayek RTX ventilator (most commonly used ventilator) which delivers the negative pressure [20].

Modes of NPV

At present NPV can be delivered via four different modes:

1) *Continuous negative expiratory pressure (CNEP)*: In this mode, the negative pressure can be maintained at a constant level throughout the respiratory cycle where the patients trigger their own breaths [21]. This is akin to NIPPV CPAP.
2) *Control or a biphasic mode*: In which a sub-atmospheric negative pressure is delivered followed by a positive (less negative) expiratory pressure. This mode provides full control over the patient's respiration, active inspiratory and expiratory phases. The provider sets up inspiratory and expiratory pressures as negative and positive numbers respectively with inspiratory: expiratory numbers 3:1 (e.g., -24, +8 cmH_2O). This mode is akin to BiPAP NIPPV as patients receive mandatory breaths at a set rate but can still take breaths in between machine breaths. Patients with chest wall deformities (e.g., kyphoscoliosis, neuro-muscular conditions like muscle dystrophies) may benefit from this mode as a result of improvement in their tidal volumes with assisted ventilation [22].
3) *Respiratory triggered*: This is a patient-triggered ventilation mode that allows for better adjustment to patient's clinical condition. The ventilator also has a backup rate set up if the patient becomes apneic. Inspiratory: expiratory ratio (I:E ratio) needs to be set by the provider.
4) *Respiratory synchronized*: In this mode, the ventilator synchronizes with the patient's breathing and automatically adjusts the respiratory rate. This mode does not need I:E ratio to be set up. There also is a backup rate similar to the respiratory triggered mode in the event of patient apnea [23].

Secretion clearance mode: This is a combination of vibration and cough modes where the ventilator can function as a chest physical therapy device. This is achieved by delivering high frequency oscillations (1200 oscillations per minute) followed by a machine generated cough which is characterized by prolonged inspiration and forced short expiration [24].

NPV Settings

The CNEP and the control (BCV) modes are the most commonly used in clinical practice. NPV is initiated in patients with acute respiratory failure with worsening respiratory status, hypoxemia, and/or hypercapnia despite maximal therapy with heated high-flow nasal cannula (HFNC) support. In a single center retrospective study, the authors described the use of NPV in pediatric acute respiratory failure not responding nor improving with HFNC support [25]. CNEP was the most used after "failure" of HFNC. In the CNEP mode, the initial pressures ranged between -8 to -16 cm H_2O.

CNEP pressures are usually adjusted in the first few minutes of initiation to achieve clinical stability with respiratory status. It is not unusual for patients to be receiving CNEP at -20 cm H_2O within the first few minutes of transitioning to NPV from HFNC.

Fraction of supplemental oxygen (FiO_2) is supplemented via the existing HFNC device to achieve SpO_2 at target range (92-97%) or via simple nasal cannula at 1-3 L/minute.

Patient's chest retractions and work of breathing can be done by visual observation through the transparent plastic cuirass shell. In addition, patient can be assessed for a "skin check" every 4-6 hours by momentarily pausing the NPV Device (i.e., RTX ventilator). This skin check examination allows the nurse, the respiratory therapist and providers to perform a cardiorespiratory and integumentary examination and decide if the CNEP support needs to be escalated or de-escalated. If escalation is needed, CNEP support is increased in increments of 2 cm H_20. Escalation of NPV means delivering "more negative" pressure to the chest wall (e.g., -20 cm H_20 is more support than -14 cm H_20). Improvement or worsening of the patient is assessed based on clinical examination: improvement respiratory rate, work of breathing, retractions, lung auscultation, or based on respiratory scoring system used in certain institutions.

Control (BCV) mode is used as an escalation from CNEP mode if no improvement or worsening of respiratory status. Inspiratory and expiratory pressure are set, usually in 3:1 ratio (e.g., -18/+6), with set respiratory rate (maximum of 60 breaths per minute) and I:E ratio of 1:1 [23].

Indications to Use NPV

Negative pressure ventilation has been used in management of hypoxemic and hypercapnic respiratory failure in several pathologies like acute respiratory distress syndrome (ARDS), bronchiolitis, pneumonia, asthma, neuromuscular conditions, and cystic fibrosis, post-operative period following Glenn and Fontan procedures.

Stone et al. used NPV in pediatric patients with acute asthma exacerbation and bronchiolitis and found improvement in patients 'overall work of breathing with the application of NPV [26]. Shum et al. looked at the safety and ease of use of negative pressure ventilation in acute bronchiolitis in pediatric patients and found that CNEP mode of NPV was safe to use and a good alternative to non-invasive positive pressure ventilation [27].

NPV has also been extensively and successfully used to treat acute hypoxemic and hypercapnic respiratory failure in patients with restrictive lung disease like chest wall deformities (e.g., kyphoscoliosis) and neuromuscular conditions (muscular dystrophies) [28].

Several studies led by Shekerdemian et al., have shown benefits of NPV on cardiac hemodynamics in the immediate post-operative period in terms of improvement in pulmonary blood flow and cardiac output in patients with tetralogy of Fallot and in immediate post-operative phase for Fontan patients. Patients with Fontan physiology have passive pulmonary blood flow, which means the pulmonary blood flow is preload dependent. Augmented negative pressure ventilation can improve venous return and thereby the pulmonary blood flow. NPV also reduces RV afterload (after proper lung recruitment and PVR reduction) and thereby improved RV stroke volume, and helps maintain lung volumes close to FRC, thus reducing pulmonary resistance and improving pulmonary blood flow [29-31].

Theoretical knowledge suggests that NPV has detrimental effects on left ventricular (LV) afterload. During NPV, inspiration causes a decrease in intra-pleural pressure and thereby increasing LV transmural pressure. This in turn increases LV afterload and hinders LV contraction. However, Chaturvedi et al. did not see this effect. They found that the use of continuous NPV in the immediate post-operative period for adults who underwent coronary artery bypass surgery improved LV stroke volume and cardiac index and improved venous return and wedge pressure [32].

Conclusion

NPV is an effective strategy to support patients with acute respiratory failure as it provides efficient ventilatory support, is well-tolerated by patients, and has favorable cardiopulmonary effects.

References

[1] Lassen H. A preliminary report on the 1952 poliomyelitis epidemic in. *Classic Papers in Critical Care.* 1953;1(1).

[2] Mehta A B, Syeda S N, Wiener R S, Walkey A J. Epidemiological trends in invasive mechanical ventilation in the United States: a population-based study. *Journal of Critical Care.* 2015;30(6):1217-21.

[3] Pierson D J. History and epidemiology of noninvasive ventilation in the acute-care setting. *Respiratory Care.* 2009;54(1):40-52.

[4] Najaf-Zadeh A, Leclerc F. Noninvasive positive pressure ventilation for acute respiratory failure in children: a concise review. *Annals of Intensive Care.* 2011; 1(1):1-10.

[5] Boldrini R, Fasano L, Nava S. Noninvasive mechanical ventilation. *Current Opinion in Critical Care.* 2012;18(1):48-53.

[6] Zimmerman J J, Rotta A T. *Fuhrman & Zimmerman's Pediatric Critical Care E-Book:* Elsevier Health Sciences; 2021.

[7] Jarrod M Mosier, John C Sakles, Sage P Whitmore, Cameron D Hypes, Danielle K Hallett, Katharine E Hawbaker, Linda S Snyder, John W Bloom . Failed noninvasive positive-pressure ventilation is associated with an increased risk of intubation-related complications. *Annals of Intensive Care.* 2015;5(1):1-9.

[8] Loring S H, Topulos G P, Hubmayr R D. Transpulmonary pressure: the importance of precise definitions and limiting assumptions. *American Journal of Respiratory and Critical Care Medicine.* 2016;194(12):1452-7.

[9] Soni N, Williams P. Positive pressure ventilation: what is the real cost? *British Journal of Anaesthesia.* 2008;101(4):446-57.

[10] Grieco DL, Chen L, Brochard L. Transpulmonary pressure: importance and limits. *Annals of Translational Medicine.* 2017;5(14).

[11] Nash G, Blen-nerhassett J B, Ponto-piddan H. RESPIRATOR LUNG SYNDROME. *Canadian Family Physician.* 1967:57.

[12] Gattinoni L, Protti A, Caironi P, Carlesso E. Ventilator-induced lung injury: the anatomical and physiological framework. *Critical Care Medicine.* 2010;38(10): S539-S48.

[13] Curley G F, Laffey J G, Zhang H, Slutsky AS. Biotrauma and ventilator-induced lung injury: clinical implications. *Chest.* 2016;150(5):1109-17.

[14] Webb H, Tierney D. Experimental pulmonary edema due to intermittent positive pressure ventilation. Protection by positive end-expiratory pressure. *Am. Rev. Respir. Dis.* 1974;110:556-65.

[15] Pressure PE-e. High inflation pressure pulmonary edema. *Am. Rev. Respir. Dis.* 1988;137:1159-64.

[16] Slutsky A S, Ranieri V M. Ventilator-induced lung injury. *The New England Journal of Medicine.* 2014;370(10):980.

[17] Mauri T., Cambhiagi B., Spinelli E., Langer T., Grasselli G., Spontaneous breathing: a double-edged sword to handle with care, *Ann. Transl. Med.* 2017;5(14):292.

[18] Mahmood S, Pinsky M. Heart-lung interactions during mechanical ventilation: the basics. *Ann. Transl. Med.* 2018;6(18):349.

[19] Thomson A., The role of negative pressure ventilation, *Archives of Disease in Childhood* 1997;77:454–458.

[20] https://www.hayekmedical.com/archives/product/hayek-rtx.

[21] Easa, D. Mundie, T.G. Finn, K.C. Hashiro, G. Balaraman, V. Continuous negative extrathoracic pressure versus positive end-expiratory pressure in piglets after saline lung lavage. *Pediatr. Pulmonol.* 1994, 17, 161–168.

[22] Kinnear, W. Hockley, S. Harvey, J.; Shneerson, J. The effects of one year of nocturnal cuirass-assisted ventilation in chest wall disease. *Eur. Respir. J.* 1988, 1, 204–208.

[23] https://buffalort.com/hayek/clinicians/modes-of-operation.

[24] Deep A. Munter C. Desai A. Negative Pressure Ventilation in Pediatric Critical Care Setting. *Indian Journal of Pediatrics,* Volume 74—May 2007.

[25] Hassinger A., Breuer R., Nutty K., Ma C-X., Al-Ibrahim A., *Negative-Pressure Ventilation in Pediatric Acute Respiratory Failure, Respiratory Care.* December 2017, vol 62, no 12.

[26] Stone R, Coddington A, Jundos R, Metz R, Whitmore J, Biphasic cuirass ventilation for respiratory distress due to asthma or bronchiolitis, *Critical Care Medicine.* 46(1):564, Jan 2018.

[27] Shum K, Al-Ibrahim O, Heard C, Biphasic cuirass ventilation use in bronchiolitis; a retrospective study, *Crit Care Med 2015,* Volume 43, Number 12 December 2015.

[28] Annunziata, A.; Calabrese, C.; Simioli, F.; Coppola, A.; Flora, M.;Marotta, A.; Di Spirito, V.; Didonna, F.; Cicalese, M.; Fiorentino, G. Negative-Pressure Ventilation in Neuromuscular Diseases in the Acute Setting. *J. Clin. Med.* 2022, 11, 2589.

[29] Shekerdemian L. S., Bush A., Shore D. F., Lincoln C., Redington A.N.: Cardiorespiratory responses to negative pressure ventilation after tetralogy of Fallot repair: a hemodynamic tool for patients with a low-output state. *J. Am. Coll. Cardiol.* 1999; 33: pp. 549-555.

[30] Shekerdemian L. S., Bush A., Shore D. F., Lincoln C., Redington A. N.: Cardiopulmonary interactions after Fontan operations: augmentation of cardiac output using negative pressure ventilation. *Circulation* 1997; 96: pp. 3934-3942.

[31] Shekerdemian L. S., Schulze-Neick I., Redington A. N., Bush A., Penny D. J.: Negative pressure ventilation as hemodynamics rescue following surgery for congenital heart disease. *Intensive Care Med.* 2000; 26: pp. 93-96.

[32] Chaturvedi R. K., Zidulka A. A., Goldberg P., deVarennes B., Iqbal S., Rahme E., Lachapelle K.: Use of negative extrathoracic pressure to improve hemodynamics after cardiac surgery. *Ann. Thorac. Surg.* 2008; 85: pp. 1355-1360.

Chapter 15

Ventilator-Induced Lung Injury in Preterm Infants

M. O'Reilly[1,2], PhD
and G. M. Schmölzer[1,2,*], MD, PhD

[1] Centre for the Studies of Asphyxia and Resuscitation,
Neonatal Research Unit, Royal Alexandra Hospital, Edmonton, Alberta, Canada
[2] Department of Paediatrics, University of Alberta, Edmonton, Alberta, Canada

Abstract

Around 10-20% of newborns (approximately 13-26 million worldwide) require respiratory support after birth. Preterm infants have structurally immature and surfactant-deficient lungs, which are not uniformly ventilated and therefore vulnerable to ventilator-induced lung injury (VILI). Invasive and non-invasive ventilation strategies applied in the delivery room, or the neonatal intensive care unit aim to maintain lung aeration and oxygenation, however, these strategies can also injure the lung and cause VILI.

Keywords: lung injury, preterm infants, mechanical ventilation, ventilator-induced lung injury, breathing

Introduction

Establishing breathing and oxygenation after birth is vital for survival and long-term health [1, 2]. While most newborn infants will successfully make

---

* Corresponding Author's Email: georg.schmoelzer@me.com.

In: Ventilator Induced Lung Injury in Non-Invasive Ventilatory Support
Editor: Antonio M. Esquinas
ISBN: 979-8-88697-840-7

the transition from fetal to neonatal life without help [3], between 10-20% of newborns (approximately 13-26 million worldwide) require non-invasive or invasive respiratory support at birth [4, 5]. Extremely preterm infants have difficulties in establishing effective breathing after birth as their lungs are structurally immature, surfactant-deficient, and not supported by a stiff chest wall [1, 2, 6].

Preterm infants are vulnerable to ventilator-induced lung injury (VILI) because their partially fluid-filled immature lungs, which are not uniformly ventilated and often surfactant-deficient. The use of ventilation strategies in the delivery room and in the neonatal intensive care unit to establish a functional residual capacity and maintain lung aeration and oxygenation, although lifesaving in many cases, can also injure the lung and cause various traumas at a cellular level. Mechanical ventilation can injure the preterm lungs and multiple ventilation strategies have been postulated to reduce VILI and improve outcomes [7].

Ventilator-Induced Lung Injury: Mechanisms

Mechanical ventilation can result in diffuse lung injury including hyaline membrane formation, interstitial and alveolar edema, hemorrhage, increased alveolar-capillary membrane permeability, impaired surfactant function, decreased lung compliance, and poor gas exchange [7-9]. Ventilator-induced inflammatory responses are responsible for some of these diffuse lung injuries, however direct cellular and tissue injury due to excessive physical force caused by regional lung over-inflation or regional lung under-inflation are further mechanisms for VILI [8, 9].

Mechanical ventilation with high tidal volumes stimulates the lung to release products (i.e., interleukin-1β (IL-1β), interleukin-6 (IL-6), interleukin-8 (IL-8), interleukin-10 (IL-10), and tumor necrosis factor alpha (TNF)-α), and mRNA levels) that promote an inflammatory cascade within 2 hours of starting ventilation as well as synthesize extracellular matrix components and growth factors [7, 10]. These cytokines and chemokines then amplify the injury response by attracting peripheral leukocytes into the lungs [7]. In comparison, ventilation with tidal volumes below functional residual capacity results in cyclic opening and closing of lung units also releases cytokines resulting in lung injury [7, 11]. Irrespective high and low lung volume ventilation resulting in either overdistension or underinflation promotes lung injury.

Barotrauma

Barotrauma was often synonymously associated with air leaks, which is the most evident macroscopic manifestation of VILI. Although, early studies demonstrated that a pressure gradient between an alveolus and its adjacent broncho vascular sheath could disrupt the pulmonary epithelium, which would allow gas to extravasate into the interstitium, mediastinum, retroperitoneum, subcutaneous tissues, or into the pleural, pericardial, or peritoneal spaces [12]. Subsequent studies reported that other factors also weaken the resilience of lung tissue including oxygen toxicity, inflammation or over-distension are also involved in the pathogenesis of air leaks [7-9, 12-15]. Further studies reported that the key determinant of this type of injury is lung overdistension, and not high airway pressures per se [7-9, 12-18].

Dreyfuss et al., ventilated rats with peak inflation pressure (PIP) at 45 cmH_2O for various time frames to assess degree of lung injury by examining lung edema and pulmonary microvascular permeability [19]. After 5 min of ventilation with high PIP, a significant increase in lung edema and pulmonary microvascular permeability when compared with control rats who were mechanically ventilated with a PIP of 7 cmH_2O [19]. The lung edema and pulmonary microvascular permeability remained almost unchanged if high PIP was applied for 10 minutes [19]. However, after 20 minutes of high PIP ventilation there was alveolar flooding and further significant increase in pulmonary microvascular permeability. In addition, anatomical damage including epithelial lesions and hyaline membranes occurred [19]. This suggests that over-inflation can cause additional damage during the ventilatory management of patients with acute respiratory failure [19].

Hernandez et al., ventilated premature rabbits with either 15, 30, and 45 cm H_2O PIP for 1 hour [16]. The lungs of premature rabbits ventilated with PIP of 15cmH_2O appeared grossly normal with pink color and no areas of hemorrhages or atelectasis [16]. With a PIP of 30cmH_2O the lungs showed a few spotty areas of hemorrhage and localized areas of atelectasis but no regions of obvious consolidation, while a PIP of 45cmH_2O resulted in grossly consolidated in the dependent regions of both lungs with localized air leaks [16]. Hernandez et al., compared these results to preterm rabbits who were covered in a full-body plaster cast to prevent lung expansion. The lungs of the preterm rabbits who were covered in a full-body plaster cast appeared completely normal with no hemorrhage, atelectasis, or areas of consolidation regardless of PIP used [16]. None of the casted animals had edema fluid in the trachea, and none developed a pneumothorax.

This data indicates that volume distension resulting in overdistension rather than high airway pressure per se result in microvascular damage in the immature lung [16].

Volutrauma

High tidal volume delivery during mechanical ventilation causes overdistention of the lung, which plays a key role in VILI. Björklund et al., reported that just 6 manual inflations with tidal volume of 30 mL/kg in preterm lambs decreased the effectiveness of subsequent surfactant treatment and resulted in increased lung injury characterized by epithelial necrosis in peripheral conducting airways, alveolar hyaline membranes, and recruitment of granulocytes to the airspaces. Furthermore, Wada et al., showed that the initiation of ventilation with high tidal volume (20 mL/kg) in preterm lambs causes structural injury to airspaces and epithelial leaks and can result in interference with surfactant function [20].

Hillman et al., showed that ventilation of preterm lambs with tidal volume of 15 mL/kg for the first 15 min of life results in a greater than 10-fold increase in protein in the bronchoalveolar lavage fluid (an indicator of lung injury), as well as elevated numbers of neutrophils and monocytes [21]. Lung tissue mRNA expression of the pro-inflammatory cytokines IL-1β, MCP-1, IL-6, IL-8 was also reported. Polglase et al., reported similar outcomes, where preterm lambs were ventilated with V_T 15 or 8 mL/kg for the first 15 min of life. Regardless of V_T, increases in bronchoalveolar lavage protein were detected, as well as injury markers in the lung tissue (increased mRNA expression of IL-1β, IL-6, IL-8, and TLR2) [22]. Hillman et al., also showed that initiation of ventilation using V_T increasing from 5 to 15 mL/kg over the first 15 min of life induced expression of a stress response and inflammatory cytokines in small and medium-sized airways, and bronchial epithelial disruption in medium-sized airways of preterm lambs [23]. Even using a lower V_T for initial ventilation (6 mL/kg during the first 15 min of life) in preterm lambs still resulted in increased expression of pro-inflammatory cytokines in the lung tissue (IL-1β, IL-6, IL-8, MCP-1, MCP-2) [24]. Inflammatory cells in the bronchoalveolar lavage were also increased, with an overall increase in the percent of monocytes [24].

Although ventilation with V_T 6 mL/kg caused less damage compared to using V_T 15 mL/kg (compared to studies by the same group, Hillman et al., [21]) as evident by no apparent airway epithelial sloughing, using low V_T of

6 mL/kg can still lead to airway stretch and lung inflammation [24]. Taken together these animal studies indicate that brief, high V_T ventilation, similar to what might occur in the delivery room during neonatal resuscitation, can initiate an injurious process in the preterm lung, suggesting that if V_T is controlled to avoid over-distension, lung injury during neonatal resuscitation may be hindered.

Biotrauma

Mechanical ventilation not only physically disrupts the lung, but it also activates and recruits inflammatory cells leading to the production of a number of inflammatory mediators (i.e., interleukins, tumor necrosis factors or mRNA), which also play a role in initiating or prolonging lung injury. The mediators are released by different mechanisms including necrosis, decompartmentalization, stretch, or shear stress [14]. The cytokine release, inflammatory cell recruitment or release of inflammatory mediators occur secondary to injuries caused by volutrauma or Atelectrauma [8].

Harling et al., examined lung inflammation marker (i.e., IL-6, IL-10, IL-1β and TNF-α) in the bronchoalveolar fluid in preterm infants who were resuscitated with either a positive pressure ventilation or sustained inflation [30]. Overall there was no difference in median (IQR) IL-6 with 6790 (104–19708) versus 1156 (42–15192) $p = 0.69$, IL-1β with 38 (5–2590) versus 43 (0–663) $p = 0.86$, IL-10 with 652 (78–1993) versus 608 (0–1242) $p = 0.67$, and TNF-α with 25 (0–1838) versus 21 (0–143) p 0.5 with either positive pressure ventilation or sustained inflation [30]. This suggests that a single lung recruitment maneuver at birth does not increase inflammatory markers 10 hours after birth. While this is reassuring, more recently sustained inflations have been associated with increased mortality and therefore should not be used during respiratory support of preterm infants [4, 5, 31, 32].

Similar, using 50% or 100% oxygen during initial resuscitation did not change increase inflammatory markers 10 hours after birth and had no influence on bronchopulmonary dysplasia or mortality [33]. Lista et al., compared synchronized intermittent positive-pressure ventilation with two different tidal volumes during the acute phase of respiratory distress syndrome. Preterm infants were randomized to be ventilated with tidal volume of 5 mL/kg or 3 ml/kg and proinflammatory cytokines including IL-6, IL-8, and TNF-α were measured on in tracheal aspirate on days 1, 3, and 7 after birth. IL-8 and TNF-α levels on day 7 were significantly higher ($p < 0.05$) and mechanical ventilation was longer in infants who were ventilated with tidal volumes of 3 mL/kg (16 ± 4 vs. 9 ± 4 days; $p = 0.05$).

This data suggests that low tidal volume ventilation causes significant higher lung inflammation in preterm infants while ventilation with tidal volumes ~5 mL/kg has a lower inflammatory response during the acute phase of respiratory distress and has a positive effect on the length of ventilation. What remains unclear is if this would prevent bronchopulmonary dysplasia.

Atelectrauma

Mechanical ventilation using low lung volume can result in atelectasis, which might lead to lung injury characterized by hyaline membrane formation, distal airway cell denudation, impaired alveolar capillary permeability, surfactant dysfunction, decreased lung compliance, and poor gas exchange [25, 26]. Several mechanisms for this "low volume" lung injury have been proposed.

Because of the repeated reopening and collapse cytokines (e.g., IL-6, IL-8, IL-1β, TNF-α) are released, which results in accumulation and activation of leukocytes within the lungs [8, 9]. The leukocyte activation is characterized by epithelial disruption, hyaline membrane formation, airway cell loss, increased alveolar capillary permeability, surfactant dysfunction, decreased lung compliance, and poor gas exchange [2, 7, 8, 13, 15, 16, 19]. Mechanical ventilation with inadequate positive end-expiratory pressure (PEEP) leads to a low residual volume and atelectasis [27, 28]. Mechanical ventilation without PEEP may lead to failure to establish functional residual capacity, inadequate oxygenation, and increasing atelectrauma [27–29].

In surfactant-treated preterm lambs, PPV without PEEP was associated with reduced compliance and oxygenation compared with ventilation with PEEP of 4 to 7 cm H_2O. In addition, preterm lambs ventilated with PEEP of 8 cm H_2O had a significantly lower oxygen requirement by 10 minutes of age compared with lambs ventilated with no PEEP. In fact, improved oxygenation has been found to occur more rapidly with PEEP than with administration of exogenous surfactant.

Conclusion

While many of the different mechanism for ventilator-induced lung injury is detailed studied in in the adult lung or newborn animals, there is a lack of data on the impact of these mechanisms on ventilator induced lung injury in the preterm human lung.

References

[1] Pas A. B. te, Davis P. G., Hooper S. B., Morley C. J. From liquid to air: breathing after birth. *J Pediatr* 2008; 152:607–11. https://doi.org/10.1016/j.jpeds.2007.10.041.

[2] Schmölzer G. M., Pas A. B. te, Davis P. G., Morley C. J. Reducing lung injury during neonatal resuscitation of preterm infants. *J Pediatr* 2008; 153:741–5. https://doi.org/10.1016/j.jpeds.2008.08.016.

[3] Aziz K., Chadwick M., Baker M., Andrews W. Ante- and intra-partum factors that predict increased need for neonatal resuscitation. *Resuscitation* 2008; 79:444–52. https://doi.org/10.1016/j.resuscitation.2008.08.004.

[4] Aziz K., Lee H. C., Escobedo M. B., Hoover A. V., Kamath-Rayne B. D., Kapadia V. S., David J. Magid, Susan Niermeyer, Georg M. Schmölzer, Edgardo Szyld, Gary M. Weiner, Myra H. Wyckoff, Nicole K. Yamada and Jeanette Zaichkin. Part 5: Neonatal Resuscitation: 2020 American Heart Association Guidelines for Cardiopulmonary Resuscitation and Emergency Cardiovascular Care. *Circulation* 2020; 142:1–27. https://doi.org/10.1161/cir.0000000000000902.

[5] Wyckoff M. H., Wyllie J. P., Aziz K., Almeida M. F. de, Fabres J., Fawke J., Ruth Guinsburg, Shigeharu Hosono, Tetsuya Isayama, Vishal S. Kapadia, Han-Suk Kim, Helen G. Liley, Christopher J. D. McKinlay, Lindsay Mildenhall, Jeffrey M. Perlman, Yacov Rabi, Charles C. Roehr, Georg M. Schmölzer, Edgardo Szyld, Daniele Trevisanuto, Sithembiso Velaphi and Gary M. Weiner. Neonatal Life Support: 2020 International Consensus on Cardiopulmonary Resuscitation and Emergency Cardiovascular Care Science With Treatment Recommendations. *Circulation* 2020; 142:329–37. https://doi.org/10.1161/cir.0000000000000895.

[6] Hooper S. B., Pas A. B. te, Kitchen M. Respiratory transition in the newborn: a three-phase process. *Archives of Disease in Childhood-Fetal*. 2016;101: F266-71. https://doi.org/10.1136/archdischild-2013-305704.

[7] Jobe A. H., Ikegami M. Mechanisms initiating lung injury in the preterm. *Early Hum Dev* 1998;53:81–94. https://doi.org/10.1016/s0378-3782(98)00045-0.

[8] Tremblay L. N., Slutsky A. S. *Ventilator-induced Injury: From Barotrauma to Biotrauma.*, 1997.

[9] Tremblay L. N., Slutsky A. S. Ventilator-induced lung injury: from the bench to the bedside. *Intensive Care Medicine* 2005; 32:24–33. https://doi.org/10.1007/s00134-005-2817-8.

[10] Berg J. T., Fu Z., Breen E. C., Tran H. C., Mathieu-Costello O., West J. B. High lung inflation increases mRNA levels of ECM components and growth factors in lung parenchyma. *J Appl Physiol* 1997; 83:120–8. https://doi.org/10.1152/jappl.1997.83.1.120.

[11] Coalson J. J., Winter V. T., Gerstmann D. R., Idell S., King R. J., Delemos R. A. Pathophysiologic, Morphometric, and Biochemical Studies of the Premature Baboon with Bronchopulmonary Dysplasia. *Am Rev Respir Dis* 1992; 145:872–81. https://doi.org/10.1164/ajrccm/145.4_pt_1.872.

[12] Macklin C. C. Transport Of Air Along Sheaths Of Pulmonic Blood Vessels From Alveoli To Mediastinum: Clinical Implications. *Arch Intern Med* 1939; 64:913–26. https://doi.org/10.1001/archinte.1939.00190050019003.

[13] Dreyfuss D., Soler P., Basset G., Saumon G. High inflation pressure pulmonary edema. Respective effects of high airway pressure, high tidal volume, and positive end-expiratory pressure. *The American Review of Respiratory Disease* 1988; 137:1159–64. https://doi.org/10.1164/ajrccm/137.5.1159.

[14] Dreyfuss D., Ricard J. D. Biotrauma hypothesis of ventilator-induced lung injury-From the authors. *American …*; 2004.

[15] Dreyfuss D., Saumon G. Barotrauma is volutrauma, but which volume is the one responsible? *Intens Care Med* 1992; 18:139–41. https://doi.org/10.1007/bf0170 9236.

[16] Hernandez L. A., Peevy K. J., Moise A. A., Parker J. C. Chest wall restriction limits high airway pressure-induced lung injury in young rabbits. *Journal of Applied Physiology* 1989; 66:2364–8. https://doi.org/10.1152/jappl.1989.66.5.2364.

[17] Dreyfuss D., Martin-Lefèvre L., Saumon G. Hyperinflation-Induced Lung Injury during Alveolar Flooding in Rats. *Am J Respir Crit Care Med.* 1999; 159:1752–7. https://doi.org/10.1164/ajrccm.159.6.9805018.

[18] Dreyfuss D., Soler P., Saumon G. Mechanical ventilation-induced pulmonary edema. Interaction with previous lung alterations. *American Journal of Respiratory and Critical Care Medicine* 1995; 151:1568–75. https://doi.org/10.1164/ajrccm. 151.5.7735616.

[19] Dreyfuss D., Basset G., Soler P., Saumon G. Intermittent positive-pressure hyperventilation with high inflation pressures produces pulmonary microvascular injury in rats. *The American Review of Respiratory Disease* 1985; 132:880–4.

[20] Wada K., Jobe A. H., Ikegami M. Tidal volume effects on surfactant treatment responses with the initiation of ventilation in preterm lambs. *Journal of Applied Physiology* (Bethesda, Md: 1985) 1997;83:1054–61.

[21] Hillman N. H., Kramer B. W., Moss T. J. M., Kallapur S. G., Bachurski C., Pillow J. J., Graeme R. Polglase, Ilias Nitsos, Boris W. Kramer, Alan H. Jobe. Brief, Large Tidal Volume Ventilation Initiates Lung Injury and a Systemic Response in Fetal Sheep. *American Journal of Respiratory and Critical Care Medicine* 2007; 176: 575–81. https://doi.org/10.1164/rccm.200701-051oc.

[22] Polglase G. R., Hillman N. H., Pillow J. J., Cheah F. C., Nitsos I., Moss T. J. M., Boris W. Kramer, Machiko Ikegami, Suhas G. Kallapur, and Alan H. Jobe. Positive End-Expiratory Pressure and Tidal Volume During Initial Ventilation of Preterm Lambs. *Pediatr Res* 2008;64:517–22. https://doi.org/10.1203/pdr.0b013e318184 1363.

[23] Hillman N. H., Kallapur S. G., Pillow J. J., Moss T. J. M., Polglase G. R., Nitsos I., Alan H. Jobe. Airway Injury From Initiating Ventilation in Preterm Sheep. *Pediatric Research* 2010;67:60–5. https://doi.org/10.1203/pdr.0b013e3181c1b09e.

[24] Hillman N. H., Moss T. J., Nitsos I., Jobe A. H. Moderate tidal volumes and oxygen exposure during initiation of ventilation in preterm fetal sheep. *Pediatric Research* 2012;72:593–9. https://doi.org/10.1038/pr.2012.135.

[25] Muscedere J. G., Mullen J. B. M., Gan K., Slutsky A. S. Tidal ventilation at low airway pressures can augment lung injury. *American Journal of Respiratory and Critical Care Medicine* 1994;149:1327–34. https://doi.org/10.1164/ajrccm.149.5.8173774.

[26] Dreyfuss D., Saumon G. *Ventilator-induced Lung Injury* 1998;157:294–323. https://doi.org/10.1164/ajrccm.157.1.9604014.

[27] Probyn M., Hooper S. B., Dargaville P. A., Mccallion N., Crossley K. J., Harding R., Colin J. Morley. Positive end expiratory pressure during resuscitation of premature lambs rapidly improves blood gases without adversely affecting arterial pressure. *Pediatric Research* 2004;56:198–204. https://doi.org/10.1203/01.pdr.0000132752.94155.13.

[28] Probyn M., Hooper S. B., Dargaville P. A., Mccallion N., Harding R., Morley C. J. Effects of tidal volume and positive end-expiratory pressure during resuscitation of very premature lambs. *Acta Paediatrica* (Oslo, Norway : 1992) 2005;94:1764–70. https://doi.org/10.1080/08035250510029 61.

[29] Hooper S. B., Siew M. L., Kitchen M. J., Pas A. B. te. Establishing functional residual capacity in the non-breathing infant. *Seminars Fetal Neonatal Medicine* 2013; 18:336–43. https://doi.org/10.1016/j.siny.2013.08.011.

[30] Harling A. E., Beresford M. W., Vince G. S., Bates M., Yoxall C. W. Does sustained lung inflation at resuscitation reduce lung injury in the preterm infant? *Archives of Disease in Childhood-Fetal* … 2005;90: F406-10. https://doi.org/10.1136/adc.2004.059303.

[31] Kirpalani H. M., Ratcliffe S. J., Keszler M., Davis P. G., Foglia E. E., Pas A. B. te, Melissa Fernando, Aasma Chaudhary, Russell Localio, Anton H van Kaam, Wes Onland, Louise S. Owen, Georg M. Schmölzer, Anup Katheria, Helmut Hummler, Gianluca Lista, Soraya Abbasi, Daniel Klotz, Burkhard Simma, Vinay Nadkarni, Francis R. Poulain, Steven M. Donn, Han-Suk Kim, Won Soon Park, Claudia Cadet, Juin Yee Kong, Alexandra Smith, Ursula Guillen, Helen G. Liley, Andrew O. Hopper, Masanori Tamura. Effect of Sustained Inflations vs Intermittent Positive Pressure Ventilation on Bronchopulmonary Dysplasia or Death Among Extremely Preterm Infants. *JAMA : The Journal of the American Medical* Association 2019; 321:1165–11. https://doi.org/10.1001/jama.2019.1660.

[32] Foglia E. E., Pas A. B. te, Kirpalani H. M., Davis P. G., Owen L., Kaam A. H. van, Wes Onland, Martin Keszler, Georg M. Schmölzer, Helmut Hummler, Gianluca Lista, Carlo Dani, Petrina Bastrenta, Russell Localio, Sarah J. Ratcliffe. Sustained Inflation vs Standard Resuscitation for Preterm Infants. *JAMA Pediatrics* 2020;174: e195897-9. https://doi.org/10.1001/jamapediatrics.2019.5897.

[33] Harling A. E., Beresford M. W., Vince G. S., Bates M., Yoxall C. W. Does the use of 50% oxygen at birth in preterm infants reduce lung injury? *Archives of Disease in Childhood-Fetal* … 2005;90:F401-5. https://doi.org/10.1136/adc.2004.059287.

Chapter 16

Management and Prevention of Ventilator Lung Injury in Children and Neonates with CPAP

Mariana Miranda[1,*], MD,
Rebecca Mitting[1], MbCHB MRCPCH
and Padmanabhan Ramnarayan[1,2], MD PhD
[1] Pediatric Intensive Care Unit, St. Mary's Hospital,
Imperial College Healthcare NHS Trust, London, UK
[2] Imperial College, London, UK

Abstract

Mechanic ventilation can cause iatrogenic ventilator-induced lung injury at any age, although the impact of ventilator-associated lung injury is particularly important in preterm neonates owing to the risk of developing bronchopulmonary dysplasia and chronic lung disease. There is no direct evidence that lung injury can be minimised by continuous positive airway pressure, nevertheless it offers the advantage of avoiding complications associated with invasive ventilation. The limited evidence which is applicable to the pediatric and neonatal population will be reviewed in this chapter.

A trial of non-invasive ventilation for most hemodynamically stable infants and children with respiratory failure, who do not require emergent intubation and lack other contraindications, is proven to be safe. However, for non-invasive ventilation to be effective and safe, patient selection, contraindications, predictors of failure, benefits and risks need to be taken into careful consideration.

* Corresponding Author's Email: mariana.miranda@nhs.net.

In: Ventilator Induced Lung Injury in Non-Invasive Ventilatory Support
Editor: Antonio M. Esquinas
ISBN: 979-8-88697-840-7

Keywords: continuous positive airway pressure ventilation, pediatric, neonatal, non-invasive ventilation, ventilator lung-induced injury

Introduction

Non-invasive ventilation (NIV) offers mainly five important physiological benefits [1-2]:

- Recruiting alveoli, increasing the functional residual capacity and decreased ventilation-perfusion (V-Q) mismatch.
- Augmenting minute ventilation.
- Maintaining airway patency, assisting the expiratory flow, and avoiding alveolar collapse.
- Decreasing work of breathing, increasing tone and contractility of the diaphragm muscles.
- Assisting left ventricular systolic function, as increasing the intrathoracic pressure reduces left ventricular transmural pressure in systole, which reduces afterload.

Continuous positive airway pressure (CPAP) can be utilized to decrease dynamic upper airway obstruction (as seen in tracheomalacia, laryngomalacia, and oropharyngeal hypotonia), work of breathing and apnea related to acute respiratory failure in infants and children. The most common example of the use of CPAP in pediatric age include infants with bronchiolitis and intermittent apnoea who benefit from the stimulation provided by NIV, or those with increased work of breathing who appear at risk of tiring.

Children with reversible obstructive processes, such as status asthmaticus or croup, or pneumonia may also benefit from CPAP, even if not hypoxic. CPAP can reduce work of breathing and hold open the airway in these patients. In asthma, theoretically by setting a positive end-expiratory pressure (PEEP) to match the intrinsic PEEP of the patient, the negative transpleural pressure needed to breathe lowers and work of breathing is reduced. This is key as 'exhaustion' is a common indication for invasive ventilation.

In the neonatal population, CPAP is widely used for respiratory support in most prematurity groups and even for prevention of respiratory distress syndrome (RDS). One of the main advantages of CPAP is that is relatively easy to use, adjust and can be delivered by trained professionals outside of intensive care setting, reducing the need to retrieve these patients from local hospitals [2-3].

Ventilator-Induced Lung Injury with CPAP

While lifesaving, any type of mechanic ventilation can cause iatrogenic ventilator-induced lung injury (VILI) at any age, making VILI prevention critical. From a physiological perspective, the inflammation and fibrosis seen in the lungs of patients who have undergone long term ventilation (> 2 weeks), is probably related to mechanical trauma and oxygen toxicity [4]. The lung was not designed to cope with high pressure ventilation or high concentration oxygen, and both can cause damage in small airways and alveoli, setting up an inflammatory reaction. Alveolar injury results in increased alveolar permeability, interstitial and alveolar edema, alveolar hemorrhage, hyaline membranes, loss of functional surfactant, and alveolar collapse, findings similar to those observed in acute respiratory distress syndrome (ARDS) [4, 5].

A clinical challenge with NIV arises when ventilator settings are minimal, yet a vigorous patient effort results in potentially self-induced harmful transpulmonary pressures and volumes during spontaneous breaths. Reversible causes of a vigorous inspiratory effort (e.g., pain, acidosis, anxiety) must be addressed and corrected.

Unfortunately, there is no direct evidence that lung injury can be minimised by NIV. However, CPAP provides the advantage of avoidance of the complications associated with invasive airway management, including avoidance of [6]:

- Airway trauma injury, aspiration, or cardiorespiratory arrest potentially during induction or difficult intubation.
- Longstanding mucosal pressure from endotracheal tube or cuff malposition, with risk of developing subglottic stenosis (especially prevalent in the ex-preterm population).
- Ventilator induced lung injury including oxygen toxicity, barotrauma, volutrauma, atelectrauma and biotrauma.
- Disruption of airway clearance mechanisms, increasing risk of ventilator-associated pneumonia and its resultant lung injury.

- Cardiopulmonary interactions leading to decreased cardiac output and increased intracranial pressure owing to decreasing venous return.
- Potential adverse effects or complications related to the need to sedate patients to facilitate invasive mechanical ventilation including the development of delirium, iatrogenic withdrawal syndrome and concerns regarding future neurodevelopmental outcomes.

Several observational and randomized studies suggest that CPAP is effective in improving ventilation, oxygenation and avoiding need for escalation of therapy during management of acute respiratory compromise in infants and children, with some studies reporting a success rate of 75 to 95% for infants with bronchiolitis and hypoxemia. However, systematic reviews have found the evidence regarding CPAP for bronchiolitis to be inconclusive because of methodologic limitations and imprecision in the existing studies [7-15]. In relation to the comparing high flow nasal cannula (HFNC) to CPAP for respiratory support in bronchiolitis, the most recent meta-analysis showed no differences in 'treatment failure' or rate of intubation, however the small sample size limits any firm conclusions regarding effectiveness [16].

The impact of VILI is particularly important in preterm neonates as bronchopulmonary dysplasia (BPD) is still the most prevalent complication related to prematurity despite developments in the treatment of RDS and is associated with substantial morbidity. The etiology of BPD is multifactorial, triggered by VILI and possible underlying infection, in a functionally immature and structurally premature lung (including poorly developed airway support structures, surfactant deficiency, decreased compliance, underdeveloped antioxidant mechanisms, and inadequate fluid clearance) [17, 18].

In the neonatal population, some interesting cohort studies and meta-analyses have shown that, in neonates with RDS, CPAP is associated with reduced mortality and need for escalation to invasive ventilation, with similar risk for BPD, when compared with supportive care with only supplemental oxygen [19]. In very preterm infants (gestational age < 32 weeks), prophylactic nasal CPAP (started within the first 15 minutes of life, before the onset of respiratory disease) has been shown to significantly reduce the incidence of BPD, the combined outcome of death and BPD, need of mechanical ventilation, and probably of pneumothorax, when compared to invasive mechanical ventilation (IMV) [20, 21]. Follow-up studies at 18 to 22 months corrected age showed the group allocated to CPAP compared with those assigned to intubation and surfactant had less respiratory morbidity and similar rates of death or neurodevelopmental impairment [22, 23].

However, extremely preterm (gestational age < 28 weeks) survivors remain at risk for impaired pulmonary function at eight years of age despite the use of CPAP. Furthermore, in preterm and very preterm infants, there is insufficient evidence to evaluate prophylactic CPAP compared to oxygen therapy and very early CPAP (started within the first hour of life), and there is no information about the effect of prophylactic or very early CPAP in late preterm infants [20, 21].

Another indication for CPAP is as rescue therapy, in patients who develop acute respiratory failure in the first 24 to 72 hours following extubation, or prophylactic, as weaning mode of respiratory support for infant's post-extubation, in patients who are at high risk of extubation failure. It reduces the incidence of adverse clinical events (apnea, respiratory acidosis, and increased oxygen requirements) and the need for reintubation [24, 25].

The recent FIRST ABC trial brought some clarity regarding the best strategy for post-extubation respiratory support in children (above 36 weeks of corrected gestational age). This trial concluded that among critically ill children requiring noninvasive respiratory support following extubation, HFNC (at 2L/kg/min) compared with CPAP (at 7-8 cmH_2O) following extubation failed to meet the criterion for noninferiority considering time to liberation from respiratory support. Furthermore, mortality at day 180 was significantly higher for HFNC [26].

Therapeutic Strategies for Prevention and Management of Ventilator-Induced Lung Injury

The therapeutic strategies to support gas exchange while minimizing lung injury are based upon the avoidance of invasive MV through preferential use of noninvasive respiratory support and applying some of the same lung protective strategies for invasive MV, including [5, 27, 28]:

- *Using a higher positive end-expiratory pressure (PEEP) strategy* to maintain lung recruitment and avoid atelectrauma. Although, the choice should be balanced, choosing the lowest possible PEEP to keep appropriate gas exchange but avoid exposure to VILI and the incidence of chronic lung disease in the vulnerable population.

Special attention should be given in case of obstructive lung diseases (e.g., asthma, bronchiolitis) where the impaired exhalation secondary to airway obstruction can significantly increase the risk of progressive hyperinflation and development of auto-PEEP. CPAP does not allow to specifically target small tidal volumes, low plateau pressure and driving pressure, as in invasive MV.

- *Avoidance of high inspired oxygen levels,* aiming Spo2 92-97% (avoid production of free oxygen radicals).
- *Allow permissive hypercapnia* if the pH remains > 7.25, to reduce increase needs of pressure/volume. However, gas exchange targets may vary depending on the condition.
- *Prone positioning* can possibly have advantages in lung recruitment in NIV, although its efficacy is only proved in invasive MV patients with severe ARDS.
- *De-escalation of settings and therapy as soon as clinically appropriate,* with need of frequent sequential clinical evaluations to determine response to treatment.
- *Exogenous surfactant replacement therapy* should be considered in preterm infants, especially for extremely preterm infants (< 28 weeks GA), as has showed to effectively reduce RDS mortality and morbidity in this age group (more information in chapter "Surfactant therapy in prevention alveolar lung injury").

The typical initial CPAP settings recommended are starting with PEEP of 5 to 8 cmH_2O, titrated up relatively quickly as needed, depending upon clinical response and patient tolerance. Normally the goal is SaO_2 > 92 to 95%, although the target for a specific patient should be determined based upon the patient's respiratory disease, comorbidities, perceived toxicity of support, and trajectory of illness. Studies show that is safe to use pressures of 8 to 10 cmH_2O, with no associated hemodynamic compromise [1, 7, 9, 10].

However, for CPAP to be safe, effective, and minimise lung injury, patient selection, contraindications, predictors of failure and risks need to be taken into careful consideration.

Patient Selection

Appropriate patient selection is essential to success of CPAP, making it essential to answer the follow 4 questions prior to the initiation of NIV.

Does the Patient Have Any Contraindications to NIV?

Table 1 presents the absolute and not absolute contraindications to NIV that need to be excluded or considered before starting this respiratory support.

Table 1. Contraindications for NIV [1, 7, 12]

Absolute contraindications
– *Need for emergent intubation* (e.g., cardiorespiratory arrest, severe respiratory distress, unstable cardiac arrhythmia). – *Need for airway protection* (e.g., epiglottitis, progressive upper airway oedema, burns). – *Inability to protect airway* (e.g., compromised bulbar function, paralysis of vocal cords, acutely impaired mental status, including patients in status epilepticus).
Relative contraindications
– *Hemodynamic instability requiring high levels of vasopressor support* (conventional ventilation should be considered to reduce metabolic demand). – *Hypoventilation/ constant apnoea.* – *Undrained pneumothorax*, although NIV is acceptable once a chest tube is in place. – *Facial or neurological surgery, trauma, or deformity* (e.g., micrognathia, Apert syndrome, Crouzon syndrome), as maintenance of a good mask seal will not be possible, or morbidity may be increased. – *Significant airway obstruction* (e.g., tracheal tumor, laryngeal mass). – *High aspiration risk* (e.g., vomiting, impaired airway protective reflexes or ability to clear secretions). – *Active upper gastrointestinal bleed.* – *Recent upper digestive tract surgery* (increased risk of dehiscence of esophageal sutures).

The decision to proceed with NIV in a patient with these conditions needs to consider the likelihood of success while weighing the potential risks of further respiratory or circulatory decompensation, which may make a later endotracheal intubation more challenging.

Is It Expected That NIV Will be Adequate to Stabilize and/or Reverse the Current Respiratory Status?

For most hemodynamically stable infants and children with hypoxemic or hypercapnic respiratory failure, who do not require emergency endotracheal intubation and lack contraindications to NIV, it is reasonable a trial of CPAP.

Table 2. Clinical conditions for which NIV could be indicated [1, 7, 29]

Acute respiratory failure	*Chronic respiratory failure*
Decompensated central nervous system diseases – Apnoea in the preterm/full-term infant. *Decompensated respiratory effort due to chest wall or spinal abnormalities* – Obesity-hypoventilation syndrome. – Chest wall trauma. *Upper airway diseases* – Laryngitis and laryngotracheitis. *Lung diseases* – Asthma. – Bronchiolitis. – Pneumonia. – Atelectasis. – Acute respiratory distress syndrome (ARDS). – Acute pulmonary oedema. *Other situations* – Post-extubation support/failure. – Peri-procedure/sedation ventilatory support. – Apnoea after tonsillectomy. – Postoperative after scoliosis corrective surgery. – Acute chest crisis. – Severe respiratory failure in palliative situation.	*Respiratory sleep disorders* – Obstructive sleep apnoea syndrome. – Primary or acquired central alveolar hypoventilation. *Neuromuscular diseases* – Disease of the 2nd motor neuron (e.g., Spinal muscular atrophy). – Diseases of/ damage of the phrenic nerve. – Myasthenia gravis and other congenital myasthenic syndromes. – Myopathies (e.g., Congenital, mitochondrial, metabolic, deposition diseases). *Upper airway diseases* – Tracheomalacia. *Respiratory diseases of the lower tract/parenchyma* – Bronchopulmonary dysplasia. – Cystic fibrosis. – Bronchiectasis.

We suggest a trial NIV should be considered early in presence of any of the following[1]:

- Moderate to severe work of breathing/ dyspnea not responsive to supplemental oxygen or other therapies (e.g., bronchodilators for status asthmaticus).
- Persistent tachypnea caused by respiratory illness.
- Hypoxemia ($FiO_2 > 0.5$ to maintain $SaO_2 > 94\%$) or mild/moderate ARDS with arterial partial pressure of oxygen (PaO_2) to FiO_2 ratio > 150 mmHg.

– Respiratory acidosis (arterial pH < 7.35 or venous pH < 7.30).

After deciding that a trial of NIV would be appropriate, it is important to consider the different types available, from CPAP, HFNC and NIV neurally adjusted ventilatory assist (NAVA).

Although still controversial, there is limited evidence that also suggests efficacy of CPAP in children with reversible obstructive processes (such as status asthmaticus or croup), pneumonia, pulmonary edema, cystic fibrosis, acute chest syndrome and dynamic upper airway obstruction (e.g., tracheomalacia, laryngomalacia, Pierre Robin syndrome) [1, 7, 29]. The full list is in Table 2.

For patients with obstructive respiratory failure with increase in respiratory muscle effort, as well as secondary retention of CO_2, NIV with two levels of pressure (bi-level positive pressure or BiPAP) tends to be more effective in improving gas exchange and reducing respiratory effort [1, 29].

Will the Patient Tolerate the Therapy?

In most children, NIV can be initiated using verbal support from parents and professionals. Nevertheless, particularly in younger children, anxiety or agitation can lead to patient-ventilator asynchrony and patients may not tolerate application of the interface or the high flow, with negative impact on effectiveness and raised risk of barotrauma.

Pharmacologic sedation might be required, however only after ensuring that hypoxia and/or hypercarbia are not the primary cause of agitation. The ideal sedative agent should provide anxiolysis without adverse impact on respiratory drive, airway protection and hemodynamic stability. Although evidence is limited, dexmedetomidine or intermittent small doses of benzodiazepines (e.g., midazolam) can be used with this purpose in intensive care settings [30].

Some data from small case series suggest that the prudent use of sedating agents does not increase the risk of need for endotracheal intubation [8]. However, patients evolving to decreased level of consciousness due to worsening hypercarbia, exhaustion, or due to effects of sedatives, will probably need invasive mechanical ventilation to protect airway.

Is There Any Identifiable Predictor of NIV Failure and What Is the Potential Risk of Complications Secondary to Failing to Protect the Airway?

Disease severity, underlying diagnosis, and inadequate response within the first one to two hours after initiation have been identified as independent predictors of NIV failure:

- *Illness severity*: Patients with high severity measured by Pediatric Risk of Mortality (PRISM) were more likely to fail NIV [31].
- *Underlying diagnosis and conditions*: Pneumonia and ARDS were identified as risk factors for NIV failure in two observational pediatric studies. Only 22% of ARDS patients treated with NIV avoided endotracheal intubation. Additionally, children with primary respiratory illness may be more likely to avoid intubation with NIV than those with conditions where prolonged ventilation might be needed, such as sepsis, malignancy, or immunosuppression. Is also influenced by comorbidities, as children that can cooperate and with better neurologic score have higher success rates [31, 32].
- *Response to treatment:* A lack of significant decline in respiratory rate, persistent high FiO_2 requirement (FiO_2 > 50% to maintain SaO_2 > 92 to 95%) and/or refractory acidosis with worsening hypercarbia (pH < 7.25) have also been identified associated with failure of NIV. Generally, significant improvement should be seen within the first two hours [10, 31, 33].

Risks and Complications of CPAP

Evidence from mostly observational studies suggest that when used in carefully selected patients with appropriate continuous monitoring, CPAP is safe for management of acute respiratory compromise across all pediatric ages [1, 29]. The decision to trial CPAP should be ultimately individual, based on clinical status, disease process and local experience.

Nevertheless, gas exchange needs may fluctuate within the same patient over time, making individualized and frequent reassessment of the adequacy of CPAP settings critical. This is particularly true in high-risk patients, as preterm neonates in the early postnatal period, when cardiorespiratory physiology changes rapidly [18, 19].

Although rare, the potential major complications of NIV also include the risk of barotrauma, self-inflicted lung injury, aspiration, hemodynamic instability, and it may delay endotracheal intubation to a time where the patient will be more instable [11, 14, 34, 35]. Another possible risk to keep in mind is that CPAP might provide insufficient PEEP if there is a large interface leak, making it inappropriate in case of undrained pneumothorax.

There are also possible minor complications that should not be ignored, as described in the Table 3. Thus, patients receiving NIV demand close monitoring and should have settings adjusted as low as possible to achieve physiologic improvement with the least amount of PEEP.

Table 3. Potential complications of NIV [11, 14, 26, 34, 35]

Major complications
– *Barotrauma* –Tension pneumothorax, pneumomediastinum, or massive subcutaneous emphysema have all occurred, with small observational studies showing rates of barotrauma from 1.4 to 9.0%, higher risk reported in low birth weight infants (birth weight < 1500 g). – *Aspiration* – Risk with higher ventilatory settings and with prophylactic attempts to decompress the stomach using a naso-gastric tube. – *Hemodynamic instability* – Depressed cardiac output due to decreasing venous return has been reported, however risk is reduced with careful selection of appropriate candidates, avoiding NIV in patients with shock that does not rapidly respond to fluid administration.
Minor complications
– *Facial skin irritation, breakdown, and ulceration* – Reported nasal/facial trauma in 5.5% of patients in recent trial. Avoided by proper mask selection (distributing pressure equally), skin protection (hydrocolloid dressing), and rotation of interface for patients enduring prolonged NIV. – *Nasal mucosal trauma* – Prevented by humidified and warmed gas delivery. – *Gastric distension* – Possible when inspiratory pressures exceed lower esophageal sphincter pressure (normally 10 mmHg) or patient swallows air (e.g., during crying), with increased the risk of aspiration. Reported in 2.6% of patients, with aspiration in 0.7%, in recent trial. – *Eye irritation or injury* – Corneal abrasion\ulceration and eye irritation or conjunctivitis, can occur if mask is in contact with the eye or with a poorly fitting mask permits air leak at the nasal bridge.

Conclusion

There is no direct evidence that lung injury can be minimised by CPAP, nevertheless CPAP offers the advantage of avoiding possible severe complications associated to invasive ventilation.

A trial of NIV for most hemodynamically stable infants and children, with hypoxemic or hypercapnic respiratory failure, who do not require emergent intubation and lack other contraindications, is proven to be safe and probably help avoiding VILI.

Potential major complications of NIV include barotrauma including air leak syndrome, aspiration, and hemodynamic instability. Careful patient selection, keeping patients calm, and frequent monitoring with frequent titration to optimize support with the lowest possible PEEP, are key for successful use of NIV and to reduce the risk of these adverse events.

Prophylactic NIV can be used especially in patients who are extubated successfully but at high risk of extubation failure, with HFNC being inferior to CPAP for this application.

References

[1] Calderini E, Chidini G, and Pelosi P. What are the current indications for noninvasive ventilation in children? *Curr. Opin. Anaesthesiol.* 2010 Jun;23(3):368-74.

[2] MacIntyre N. Physiologic Effects of Noninvasive Ventilation. *Respir. Care* 2019;64(6):617–628.

[3] Akingbola O A, Hopkins R L. Pediatric noninvasive positive pressure ventilation. *Pediatr. Crit. Care Med.* 2001 Apr;2(2):164-9.

[4] Slutsky A S, Ranieri V M. Ventilator-induced lung injury. *N. Engl. J. Med.* 2013 Nov;369(22):2126-36.

[5] Brochard L, Slutsky A, Pesenti A. Mechanical Ventilation to Minimize Progression of Lung Injury in Acute Respiratory Failure. *Am. J. Respir. Crit. Care Med.* 2017; 195:438.

[6] Hatch L D, Grubb P H, Lea A S, Walsh W F, Markham M H, Whitney GM, Slaughter JC, Stark AN, Ely EW. Endotracheal Intubation in Neonates: A Prospective Study of Adverse Safety Events in 162 Infants. *J. Pediatr.* 2016; 168:62.

[7] Abadesso C, Nunes P, Silvestre C, Loureiro H, Almeida H. Non-invasive ventilation in acute respiratory failure in children. *Pediatr. Rep.* 2012; 4:e16.

[8] Lazner M R, Basu A P, Klonin H. Non-invasive ventilation for severe bronchiolitis: analysis and evidence. *Pediatr. Pulmonol.* 2012; 47:909.

[9] Cavari Y, Sofer S, Rozovski U, Lazar I. Noninvasive positive pressure ventilation in infants with respiratory failure. *Pediatr. Pulmonol.* 2012; 47:1019.

[10] Essouri S, Chevret L, Durand P, Haas V, Fauroux B, Devictor D. Noninvasive positive pressure ventilation: five years of experience in a pediatric intensive care unit. *Pediatr. Crit. Care Med.* 2006; 7:329.

[11] Yañez L J, Yunge M, Emilfork M, Lapadula M, Alcántara A, Fernández C, Lozano J, Contreras M, Conto L, Arevalo C, Gayan A, Hernández F, Pedraza M, Feddersen M, Bejares M, Morales M, Mallea F, Glasinovic M, Cavada G. A prospective, randomized, controlled trial of noninvasive ventilation in pediatric acute respiratory failure. *Pediatr. Crit. Care Med.* 2008; 9:484.

[12] James C S, Hallewell C P, James D P, Wade A, Mok Q Q. Predicting the success of non-invasive ventilation in preventing intubation and re-intubation in the pediatric intensive care unit. *Intensive Care Med.* 2011; 37:1994.

[13] Ganu S S, Gautam A, Wilkins B, Egan J. Increase in use of non-invasive ventilation for infants with severe bronchiolitis is associated with decline in intubation rates over a decade. *Intensive Care Med.* 2012; 38:1177.

[14] Morris J V, Ramnarayan P, Parslow R C, Fleming S J. Outcomes for Children Receiving Noninvasive Ventilation as the First-Line Mode of Mechanical Ventilation at Intensive Care Admission: A Propensity Score-Matched Cohort Study. *Crit. Care Med.* 2017; 45:1045.

[15] Jat K R, Mathew J L. Continuous positive airway pressure (CPAP) for acute bronchiolitis in children. *Cochrane Database of Systematic Reviews* 2019, Issue 1. Art. No.: CD010473.

[16] Zhao X, Qin Q, Zhang X. Outcomes of High-Flow Nasal Cannula Vs. Nasal Continuous Positive Airway Pressure in Young Children with Respiratory Distress: A Systematic Review and Meta-Analysis. *Front. Pediatr.* 2021 Nov 5;9:759297.

[17] Jensen E A, Schmidt B. Epidemiology of bronchopulmonary dysplasia. *Birth Defects Res. A Clin. Mol. Teratol.* 2014; 100:145.

[18] Fischer H S, Bührer C. Avoiding endotracheal ventilation to prevent bronchopulmonary dysplasia: a meta-analysis. *Pediatrics* 2013; 132:e1351.

[19] Ho J J, Subramaniam P, Davis P G. Continuous positive airway pressure (CPAP) for respiratory distress in preterm infants. *Cochrane Database Syst. Rev.* 2020; 10:CD002271.

[20] Subramaniam P, Ho J J, Davis P G. Prophylactic, or very early initiation of continuous positive airway pressure (CPAP) for preterm infants. *Cochrane Database of Systematic Reviews 2021*, Issue 10. Art. No.: CD001243.

[21] Kanbar L J, Shalish W, Latremouille S, Rao S, Brown K A, Kearney R E, & Sant'Anna G M. Cardiorespiratory behavior of preterm infants receiving continuous positive airway pressure and high flow nasal cannula post extubation: randomized crossover study. *Pediatr. Res.* 2020; 87:62.

[22] Stevens T P, Finer N N, Carlo W A, Szilagyi P G, Phelps D L, Walsh M C, Gantz M G, Laptook A R, Yoder B A, Faix R G, Newman J E, Das A, Do B T, Schibler K, Rich W, Newman N S, Ehrenkranz R A, Peralta-Carcelen M, Vohr B R, Wilson-Costello D E, Yolton K, Heyne R J, Evans P W, Vaucher Y E, Adams-Chapman I, McGowan E C, Bodnar A, Pappas A, Hintz S R, Acarregui M J, Fuller J, Goldstein

R F, Bauer C R, O'Shea T M, Myers G J, Higgins R D. Respiratory outcomes of the surfactant positive pressure and oximetry randomized trial (SUPPORT). *J. Pediatr.* 2014; 165:240.

[23] Doyle L W, Carse E, Adams A M, Ranganathan S, Opie G, Cheong J L Y; Victorian Infant Collaborative Study Group. Ventilation in Extremely Preterm Infants and Respiratory Function at 8 Years. *N. Engl. J. Med.* 2017; 377:329.

[24] Bamat N, Fierro J, Mukerji A, Wright C J, Millar D, Kirpalani H. Nasal continuous positive airway pressure levels for the prevention of morbidity and mortality in preterm infants. *Cochrane Database of Systematic Reviews 2021*, Issue 11. Art. No.: CD012778.

[25] Sweet D G, Carnielli V, Greisen G, Hallman M, Ozek E, Te Pas A, Plavka R, Roehr C C, Saugstad O D, Simeoni U, Speer C P, Vento M, Visser G H A, Halliday H L. European Consensus Guidelines on the Management of Respiratory Distress Syndrome – 2019 Update. *Neonatology* 2019;115:432–450.

[26] Ramnarayan P, Richards-Belle A, Drikite L, Saull M, Orzechowska I, Darnell R, Sadique Z, Lester J, Morris K P, Tume L N, Davis P J, Peters M J, Feltbower R G, Grieve R, Thomas K, Mouncey P R, Harrison D A, Rowan K M; FIRST-ABC Step-Down RCT Investigators and the Paediatric Critical Care Society Study Group. Effect of High-Flow Nasal Cannula Therapy vs Continuous Positive Airway Pressure Following Extubation on Liberation from Respiratory Support in Critically Ill Children: A Randomized Clinical Trial. *JAMA*. Published online April 7, 2022.

[27] The Pediatric Acute Lung Injury Consensus Conference Group. Pediatric Acute Respiratory Distress Syndrome: Consensus Recommendations from the Pediatric Acute Lung Injury Consensus Conference. *Pediatr. Crit. Care Med.* 2015 June; 16(5): 428–439.

[28] Donlan M, Fontela P S, Puligandla P S. Use of continuous positive airway pressure (CPAP) in acute viral bronchiolitis: a systematic review. *Pediatr. Pulmonol.* 2011; 46:736.

[29] Najaf-Zadeh A, Leclerc F. Noninvasive positive pressure ventilation for acute respiratory failure in children: a concise review. *Ann. Intensive Care* 2011; 1:15.

[30] Venkatraman R, Hungerford J L, Hall M W, Moore-Clingenpeel M, Tobias J D. Dexmedetomidine for Sedation During Noninvasive Ventilation in Pediatric Patients. *Pediatr. Crit. Care Med.* 2017; 18:831.

[31] Dohna-Schwake C, Stehling F, Tschiedel E, Wallot M, Mellies U. Non-invasive ventilation on a pediatric intensive care unit: feasibility, efficacy, and predictors of success. *Pediatr. Pulmonol.* 2011; 46:1114.

[32] Marohn K, Panisello J M. Noninvasive ventilation in pediatric intensive care. *Curr. Opin. Pediatr.* 2013; 25:290.

[33] Muñoz-Bonet J I, Flor-Macián E M, Brines J, Roselló-Millet P M, Cruz Llopis M, López-Prats J L, Castillo S. Predictive factors for the outcome of noninvasive ventilation in pediatric acute respiratory failure. *Pediatr. Crit. Care Med.* 2010; 11: 675.

[34] Mayordomo-Colunga J, Medina A, Rey C, Concha A, Menéndez S, Arcos M L, Vivanco-Allende A. Non-invasive ventilation in pediatric status asthmaticus: a prospective observational study. *Pediatr. Pulmonol.* 2011; 46:949.

[35] Carroll C L, Zucker A R. Barotrauma not related to type of positive pressure ventilation during severe asthma exacerbations in children. *J. Asthma* 2008; 45:421.

Chapter 17

Surfactant Therapy in Prevention of Lung Injury in Neonates

Erika Pineda[1], MD
Hari Gourabathini[2], MD
and Omar Alibrahim[3,4,*], MD

[1] Oishei Children's Hospital, University of Buffalo,
Department of Pediatrics, Division of Pediatric Critical Care Medicine,
Buffalo, New York, USA
[2] Beacon Children's Hospital Beacon Health System, South Bend, Indiana, USA
[3] Duke University Medical Center, Durham, North Carolina, USA
[4] Duke Children's Hospital, Department of Pediatrics,
Division of Pediatric Critical Care Medicine, Durham, North Carolina, USA

Abstract

Lung development begins at approximately 26 days of gestation and continues throughout the first 36 months postnatally. Pulmonary surfactant is a lipoprotein that reduces alveolar surface tension facilitating alveolar expansion, prevents atelectasis and regulates lung inflammation. Lung immaturity in the neonate, causes decreased quantity and quality of surfactant leading to respiratory distress syndrome (RDS).

Pediatric pulmonary hemorrhage and pediatric acute respiratory distress syndrome (PARDS) can lead to alveolar influx of proteinaceous edema and inflammatory products inactivate surfactant leading to decrease in the quantity and quality. In the absence of surfactant there is alveolar collapse, decreased compliance and significant V/Q mismatching. In clinical practice, exogenous surfactant therapy is

* Corresponding Author's Email: omar.alibrahim@duke.edu.

In: Ventilator Induced Lung Injury in Non-Invasive Ventilatory Support
Editor: Antonio M. Esquinas
ISBN: 979-8-88697-840-7

available as a bolus administered intratracheally or as an aerosolized. Side effects are transient and include hypoxia, bradycardia and hypotension. Pulmonary hemorrhage and pneumothorax are reported less frequently.

Exogenous surfactant in RDS decreases the incidence of pulmonary interstitial emphysema, bronchopulmonary dysplasia, and mortality in preterm infants. In term infants with MAS, surfactant improves oxygenation and decreases severity of pulmonary morbidity. In older children with PARDS, surfactant is a potential therapeutic intervention, however, studies have provided mixed results on its benefits.

Limitations in effective surfactant dosing and delivery, phospholipase A2 inactivation of surfactant, and wrongful trial designs contribute to the lack of conclusive results. Studies considering current definitions of PARDS in randomized trials evaluating efficacy of dose with similar types of surfactants and routes of administration are necessary.

Keywords: mechanical ventilation, PARDS, surfactant, positive pressure ventilation, acute respiratory failure

Lung Development

Lung development occurs in stages, starting at approximately 26 days of gestation. During this embryonic period, the main and segmental bronchi start to develop from a ventral bud off the esophagus. From 5 to 16 weeks of gestation the airway continues to branch from the main segmental bronchi in the pseudoglandular stage. The canalicular stage occurs from 16 to 25 weeks of gestation and it is during this period that differentiation of the respiratory epithelium into type I and type 2 epithelial cells, occurs. Type II epithelial cells are the source of surfactant production [1]. This stage is followed by the saccular stage characterized by formation of large and primitive forms of alveoli. At 36 weeks of gestation alveolarization (formation of alveoli) begins in a process that continues throughout the first 36 months postnatally [2].

Prior to birth the lungs are filled with fluid and provide no respiratory function. At the time of birth, the lungs transition to providing gas exchange via repetitive inspiratory and expiratory cycles. This process occurs by hydraulic and diffusive transport mechanisms. The tracheobronchial tree, from the trachea to the terminal bronchioles, generations 0 to 16, are known as dead space with no gas exchange. Whereas generations 17 to 23, from the respiratory bronchioles to the alveolar sacs are the transitional and respiratory zones with diffuse gas exchange. Alveoli are thin-walled structures with an inner surface responsible for maximizing gas exchange and is the basic gas exchange unit. There inner area is lined with type I and type II epithelial cells. Surfactant, produced by type II epithelial cells, forms a film over the inner area of the alveolus to reduce surface tension and facilitate respiration.

Physiology of Surfactant

The air-liquid interface in the inner area of the alveoli causes differences in the attractive forces of the molecules in the region, leading to surface tension, which unopposed resists expansion of the alveoli and supports collapse. Surfactant is complex mixture composed of 90% lipids, mostly dipalmitoylphosphatidylcholine (DPPC), and ten percent proteins, responsible for reducing alveolar surface tension to facilitate alveolar expansion and reduce the likelihood of atelectasis. The tight intermolecular packing of DPPC, is thought to be largely responsible for the ability of surfactant to reduce surface tension. Surfactant lipids have also been recognized as key regulators of lung inflammation and biosensors of oxidative stress [3].

Four surfactant-specific proteins, SP-A, SP-B, SP-C, SP-D, have been identified and their functions have been partly elucidated [4]. The expression of the four surfactant proteins varies with gestational age, from SP-A at 32 weeks of gestation to SP-D in late gestation. SP-B and SP-C are hydrophobic proteins that aid in the absorption of lipids and spreading of phospholipids in the inner surface of the alveoli. In animal studies, it was found that animals with antibodies to SP-B develop respiratory failure. In humans, homozygous SP-B deficiency, although extremely rare, has a poor prognosis [5].

Further studies of peptides synthesized from the sequences of SP-B amino acids showed a cohesiveness to phospholipid molecules, leading to the theory that SP-B induces lateral stability. It has been proposed that by this mechanism, surfactant lowers and varies surface tension with the changing surface area in the stable alveolus [6]. The SP-C protein is known to cause development of interstitial lung disease and emphysema in deficient mice as they age but normal lungs and surfactant function at birth. This is similar in humans where SP-C deficiency causes progressive interstitial pulmonary fibrosis in infancy and early childhood. [7]. SP-A and SP-D are hydrophilic proteins functioning as innate host defense proteins and regulators of inflammation in the lungs [8].

Although SP-A is low in preterm lungs, it does not seem to have a critical role in the regulation of surfactant metabolism, given that studies in mice lacking this protein had normal lung function and metabolism [9]. SP-D binds pathogens and facilities their clearance.

In one animal study, preterm lambs treated with recombinant surfactant protein D inhibited lung inflammation and reduced surfactant inactivation [9]. Several other proteins are known to have a role in the production of functional surfactant including, ABCA3 (member A3 of the ATP binding cassette family of proteins) a transmembrane protein of lamellar bodies, organelles responsible for assembly and storage of surfactant, and TTF-1 (thyroid transcription factor-1 a transcription factor involved in genes encoding of ABCA3, SP-B, and SP-C to regulate their expression. The complex mixture of lipids and proteins composing surfactant play a critical role in reducing surface tension in the alveolus and modulating various aspects of innate host defense of the lung against diverse pulmonary pathogens.

Pulmonary surfactant is synthesized and assembled in the lamellar bodies of type II epithelial cells. From there it is transported and secreted into the alveolus. The compression and expansion of the alveoli with each respiratory cycle causes surfactant transformation from large, highly surface active to less active [10]. At this point, type II cells, macrophages and the alveolar lining act to degrade and recycle surfactant. This process of surfactant metabolism is slower in newborns (especially those born prematurely).

Mechanisms and Types of Lung Injury

Pulmonary surfactant reduces surface tension, even at low volumes, leading to a decrease in the required pressure, thus maintaining alveolar volume and stability. Disorders in the surfactant system may occur by disrupting the functions of proteins essential for homeostasis or from direct alveolar injury, causing proteinaceous edema and inflammatory products, which increase the conversion rate of surfactant into its inactive form. Similarly, oxidative stress and mechanical ventilation with high tidal volumes and lack of positive end-expiratory pressure (PEEP) can inactivate surfactant via mechanical stress. Furthermore, abnormal fluid absorption results in inefficient clearing of liquid in the injured lung, aggravating deficient gas exchange.

Diseases causing increased surface tension from reduced and/or absent surfactant or inactivated surfactant led to atelectasis or alveolar collapse. Generally, the smaller alveoli are more prone to collapse due to the relationship described by Laplace. However, when alveolar collapse occurs throughout the lung it causes diffuse atelectasis leading to low lung volume (functional residual capacity) and decreased compliance. There is also significant V/Q mismatch with intrapulmonary right-to-left shunting causing hypoxemia.

The most common cause of surfactant deficiency is preterm delivery [11]. Respiratory distress syndrome (RDS) is a significant cause of morbidity in preterm neonates, with a slightly male predominance [12]. Although, the primary abnormality in RDS in surfactant deficiency there is also decreased quality of surfactant secondary to lung immaturity. Lower surfactant production is seen with decreasing gestational age. In preterm infants with RDS, the surfactant pool is reduced to less than 10 mg/kg compared with term infants who have an estimated pool size of 100 mg/kg. The quality of surfactant also varies among preterm and term infants.

In a study comparing the ratio of lipids in surfactant from immature lungs with surfactant from mature lungs, the immature lung contained more amounts of phosphatidylinositol and less amounts of phosphatidylglycerol. Phosphatidylglycerol is present in higher contents in mature surfactant and has greater surface activity; it is used as a marker for fetal lung maturity. In addition, the protein to lipid ratio in preterm lungs is lower. All these factors cause minimal surface tensions to be higher for surfactant in preterm infants.

The pathogenesis of RDS involves surfactant deficiency as well as inflammation and lung injury causing inactivation of the remaining surfactant. In animal experiments of RDS, there is rapid accumulation of neutrophils and pulmonary edema and depletion of neutrophils prevented pulmonary edema [13]. Atelectasis caused by surfactant deficiency leads to respiratory epithelial and capillary endothelial injury, triggering a cytokine-mediated inflammatory response which causes further accumulation of protein-rich pulmonary fluid and deactivation of surfactant [14]. The administration of glucocorticoids antenatally reduces the risk of RDS by enhancing maturational changes in lung architecture and inducing enzymes that stimulate phospholipid synthesis and surfactant release. Corticosteroids are also known to increase levels of SP-A. Postnatally, surfactant replacement therapy reduces the incidence, morbidity and mortality associated with RDS. It is the standard of care in management of preterm infants with RDS.

Meconium aspiration syndrome (MAS) and pulmonary hemorrhage both cause inactivation of surfactant. *In vitro*, aspiration of meconium destroys the fibrillary structure of surfactant and interferes with its surface adsorption [15]. Additionally, phospholipase-A2 (PLA2) found in meconium inhibits the activity of surfactant by competitive displacement of surfactant from the alveolar film, in a dose-dependent manner. [16]. PLA2 also damages the alveolar-capillary membrane, induces an intrapulmonary inflammatory response and hydrolyzes DPPC causing surfactant dysfunction [17]. Similarly, in pulmonary hemorrhage there is extravasation of blood from increased permeability of the alveolar-capillary barrier (lung capillary pressure, fluid overload, congestive heart failure) or direct trauma. This leads to passage of hemoglobin, RBC lipids and plasma proteins into the alveolar space causing inactivation of surfactant [18].

Acute respiratory distress syndrome (ARDS) is characterized by increased permeability of the alveolar-capillary barrier from injury to the endothelium and/or alveolar epithelial cells. This causes influx of protein rich fluid to the alveoli (non-cardiogenic pulmonary edema) with decreased fluid clearance. Epithelial cells are further damaged by influx of neutrophil-derived enzymes and cytokines. This impairs gas exchange and decreases static lung compliance. In children, diagnostic criteria for pediatric respiratory distress syndrome (PARDS) were first established by the Pediatric Acute Lung Injury Consensus Conference (PALICC) in 2015. The definition of PARDS includes patients with lung disease not related to the perinatal age, acute onset of symptoms (within 7 days of a known insult), non-cardiogenic pulmonary edema (permeability pulmonary edema), chest x-ray findings of new infiltrates. PARDS has been associated to infectious processes such as pneumonia and sepsis, hemorrhage, or other forms of direct lung injury.

Permeability pulmonary edema, from alveolar epithelial and vascular endothelial injury, is the most prominent feature of ARDS. The inflammatory process that ensues leads to the presence of immune cells, including neutrophils and macrophages, inflammatory mediators, protein-rich fluid, and cellular debris [19]. A study was conducted using mathematical models of lung mechanics describing time-varying alveolar compliance in patients with ARDS shows that surfactant concentration has a strong impact on lung mechanics variables [20]. The proteins and inflammatory mediators affect the quantity and quality of surfactant. The damage caused to type II epithelial cells leads to decreased surfactant production. In addition, the hypoxemia and free radical production that occurs causes a decrease in surfactant precursors into the lung tissue. The quality of surfactant produced is also inadequate with altered lipid and protein composition.

In contrast to RDS, bronchoalveolar lavage studies in patients with ARDS shows an increase in the total protein to phospholipid ratio. Lower DPPC levels alter the capability of surfactant to reduce surface tension. Although the protein to phospholipid ratio is lower, protein concentration is also lower in surfactant of patients with ARDS, this is thought to be related to impaired synthesis at the cellular level. *In vitro* study, analyzing the effect of neutrophil elastase on surfactant activity found a marked-concentration dependent slowing of adsorption associated with proteolytic cleavage of SP-A and lower concentrations of SP-B and SP-C [21]. A study *in vivo* also shows that SP-A is cleaved by neutrophil elastase present in pulmonary edema of patients with ARDS [22]. In adults, SP-D is increased in patients with ARDS and those mechanically ventilated with high tidal volumes, serving as a marker of alveolar epithelial injury.

Similarly, a retrospective analysis involving patients across 5 PICUs found that plasma SP-D is a marker of PARDS severity and an early predictor of mortality [23]. Lung injury in ARDS further impacts the remaining surfactant complexes by inactivating its functional properties. Surfactant phospholipids are unable to bind normally due to the circulating plasma proteins (albumin and fibrinogen) which compete to bind the air-liquid interface. Qualitative and quantitative deficiency of surfactant has a role in the development of PARDS. Furthermore, surfactant dysfunction is correlated with mortality and length of PICU stay [24].

Pulmonary surfactant dysfunction related to genetic disorders occurs when there is variation in DNA sequences of genes encoding proteins critical for the production and function of surfactant. Histological findings guide the diagnoses of interstitial lung disease (ILD) in adults. In children this includes congenital alveolar proteinosis, desquamative interstitial pneumonitis (DIP), chronic pneumonitis of the infancy, nonspecific interstitial pneumonitis, and usual interstitial pneumonitis. However, genetic mechanisms that alter surfactant production and metabolism can cause DIP, as well as patterns of PAP and chronic pneumonitis of infancy [25].

Pulmonary alveolar proteinosis (PAP) is a rare lung disease, characterized by accumulation of lipoproteinaceous material within the alveoli. This can occur secondary to genetic or acquired causes. Genetic PAP, although uncommon, causes respiratory failure in newborns. Abnormal sequence variants in the genes encoding the receptor for granulocyte-macrophage colony-stimulating factor (GM-CSF) affect surfactant catabolism [26, 27]. This affects to uptake and recycling of surfactant components by alveolar macrophages thus preventing the clearance of surfactant materials, resulting in their accumulation in the alveolar air spaces.

Other genetic causes of PAP in children involve association with sequence variants of the genes SLC7A7 (resulting in the disorder lysinuric protein intolerance), MARS (encoding methionyl-tRNA synthetase), GATA2 (a transcription factor) and OAS1 [28]. Finally, specific mutations affecting SP-B and SP-C [5, 7, 29] and ABCA3 [30], have also been described [30, 31].

In clinical practice, several preparations of surfactant are available that are either animal derived or synthetic derived protein formulations. Animal derived preparations (e.g., calfactant, bovactant, bovine lipid extract surfactant, poractant alfa and beractant) are obtained through lavage or centrifugation of minced bovine or porcine lung tissue. Poractant alfa has highest concentration of SP-B and phospholipids. This allows administration of same number of phospholipids with a lower dose of poractant alfa 1. A large retrospective study showed poractant alfa therapy for RDS in preterm infants decreased mortality compared to beractant and calfactant. In comparison study of various animal derived surfactants, established beractant had significant increase in mortality prior to discharge, death or oxygenation need at 36 weeks of post menstrual age, PDA demanding treatment, intraventricular hemorrhage and receiving > 1dose of surfactant compared to poractant alfa.

In pediatric population, previous studies demonstrated improvement in oxygenation and other long-term outcomes including decreased mortality after the administration of bovine natural surfactant, calfactant (Infasurf; ONY Pharmaceuticals, Amherst, NY), in children with PARDS [32-34].

Gregory et al. reported improved oxygenation in a subgroup of adults with sepsis-induced ALI/ARDS using a natural surfactant (beractant, Survanta) [35]. A larger randomized controlled trial (RCT) using a recombinant surfactant containing surfactant protein C (Venticute) demonstrated improved oxygenation but no overall improvement in outcomes

Modes of Surfactant Delivery

Surfactant is delivered as a bolus by intratracheal instillation through endotracheal tube, bronchoscopy instillation, laryngeal mask, angiocath or feeding tube in trachea. It can be delivered through aerosolized form as well.

Adequate and appropriate first dose is vital in response to surfactant. A large meta-analysis demonstrated poractant alfa 200 mg/kg administration was associated with decreased ventilator days and adverse effects on lungs, lower incidence of BPD mortality and BPD [36]. A higher first dose decreases the need for repeated doses. Repeated doses are recommended for infants with worsening respiratory distress [37, 38]. Poractant alfa seems to have higher dose of phospholipids which might have led to it increased efficacy.

Randomized trials comparing the dose-to-dose efficacy of animal derived surfactants to establish the efficacy are needed [39].

Synthetic Surfactants

A synthetic surfactant decreases the immunological and infectious exposure risk to animal derived mammalian surfactants. It also adds more predictability and consistent concentration. Lucinactant is a peptide analog mirroring SP-B, in a phospholipid mixture nearer to human surfactant composition. Lucinactant compared to animal derived poractant alfa and beractant established safety and equivalent efficacy to animal derived surfactants [40, 41]. Lucinactant currently under development aerosolized surfactant *Aerosurf* which is undergoing pre-clinical trials.

Recombinant surfactant protein C based surfactant administration in adults with ARDS resulted in improvement of gas exchange during 24 hr. period but no benefit in survival [42].

Surfactant Therapy in Children and Adolescents

Surfactant is considered as a potential early therapeutic intervention to reverse the surfactant dysfunction in early phase of ARDS to improve gaseous exchange, improve lung compliance by recruiting more alveoli, facilitating better gas exchange, and may aid in decreasing the aggressive respiratory support [43].

Bovine surfactant instillation improved oxygenation in mild to moderate ARDS children, pulmonary mechanics, increased surfactant protein A connate in tracheal aspirate, decreased duration on ECMO and decrease in aggressive ventilation associated adverse effects [43, 44].

Early calfactant administration in infants, children, and adolescents with acute respiratory failure improved oxygenation acutely and decreased mortality significantly. There was no notable change was observed in number of ventilation days and hospital stay but mortality was unaffected. Transient hypoxia and hypotension were observed commonly with calfactant administration [44]. Calfactant administration in children with leukemia or lymphoma or post hematopoietic cell transplantation with PARDS requiring mechanical ventilation did not improve oxygenation or mortality, duration of mechanical ventilation [45]. Another study established no benefit in oxygenation and mortality with surfactant administration in children with ARDS from direct lung injury [46].

Lucinactant is a synthetic non animal derived protein which mimics surfactant protein B. It is resistant to inactivation by plasma proteins, oxidant species and carries important modulation of pulmonary inflammatory response. Intra-tracheal administration of the lucinanctant in mechanically ventilated infants with acute hypoxemic respiratory failure improved oxygenation with low side effect profile. It did not decrease the duration of mechanical ventilation. One study demonstrated decrease in the duration of mechanical ventilation days in children with less severe lung disease on administration which may be due to anti-inflammatory properties. Peri-dosing desaturations and bradycardia were transient and prevalent but not associated with unfavorable clinical outcomes [47].

Surfactant Therapy in Neonates

Surfactant therapy for neonatal RDS has proven to decrease the incidence of pneumothorax, pulmonary interstitial emphysema, bronchopulmonary dysplasia, and mortality in preterm infants. Repeated administration of surfactant boluses lead to enhancements in oxygenation and ventilator needs, diminished risk of pneumothorax and inclination to improvement of survival. Early rescue surfactant treatment (< 2 hours of age) in preterm infants with RDS decreases mortality, chronic lung disease, and air leak syndromes. Early initiation of CPAP with subsequent surfactant administration in extremely premature infants decreases incidence of BPD/death in comparison to prophylactic surfactant therapy alone [48].

Early surfactant therapy within 6 hours after birth in term infants with Meconium aspiration syndrome (MAS) improves oxygenation and decreases severity of pulmonary morbidity, and hospitalization duration [49]. Surfactant therapy in MAS decrease the severity of pulmonary illness and risk of progressive respiratory failure requiring ECMO [50]. Surfactant therapy in congenital diaphragmatic hernia had no significant outcome established. Antenatal steroids with surfactant therapy independently and adjunctively reduce mortality, severity of RDS and air leak syndromes [51].

Nebulization of surfactant via vibrating membrane in very and moderate preterm infants with mild RDS may promote successful establishment of non –invasive respiratory support by reducing the risk of intubation in certain subgroup of infants [52]. Another study revealed no difference was observed in need for mechanical ventilation and ventilation days or continuous positive pressure days [53]. Nebulization of surfactant in animal studies revealed improvement in V/Q mismatch, less adverse effects compared to direct instillation, improves homogeneity of surfactant distribution, lung compliance, and oxygenation [54].

Surfactant Therapy in ECMO

A single center retrospective study revealed improved lung compliance with surfactant administration during ECMO [55]. A similar study in cardiac patients showed improved lung compliance and function with less adverse effects reported like pulmonary hemorrhage. However, there was no significant benefit in length of stay or survival [56]. One retrospective study demonstrated improvement of lung volumes and pulmonary function resulting in weaning ECMO parameters [57]. Animal studies with surfactant administration in Pigs with severe ARDS on ECMO revealed no change in oxygenation and pulmonary functions [58].

Surfactant as a Biomarker for ARDS

Surfactant protein A (SP-A) & Surfactant protein D (SP-D) play a vital role in airway homeostasis, innate immunity, and inflammatory response in lungs and to variety of infection. Surfactant protein A & D (SP-D) part of collectin family and host innate defense system. SP-A&D increased in response to lung injury or infection. SP- A, D aids in phagocytosis of microorganisms by binding to oligosaccharides on the surface and modulated innate immunological response in lung [59, 60]. SP-D is a good marker of severity of epithelial injury and ARDS in adults.

Elevated SP-D levels in umbilical cord and capillary blood on day one in premature infants designate development of RDS and vulnerability to infection [61]. Elevated serum or plasma SP-D levels reported in adults and pediatric ARDS. SP-D in adult ARDS is associated with poor outcomes. Elevated SP-D levels is associated with severe PARDS, increased mortality, elevated oxygenation index, days on mechanical ventilation and length of stay at PICU in children with acute respiratory failure [62].

In general, studies have demonstrated relative depletion of surfactant proteins and increase in the plasma levels points towards increased permeability of alveolar capillary barrier due to direct injury or inflammation. Further studies and analysis of these markers in tracheal aspirates, bronchoalveolar lavage fluids, and plasma levels is needed in evaluating risk, replacement, and management strategies [63].

Adverse Effects

Transient hypoxia may be secondary to blockage of endotracheal tube in preterm neonates. Transient bradycardia and hypotension associated with administration are brief and well tolerated. In animal and human studies, it is speculated that surfactant has pharmacological effect on vasodilation. Mean arterial pressure decreases with administration of surfactant in dose dependent manner which is partially compensated with increase in cardiac output. The effect of increased $PaCO_2$ causing cerebral vasodilatation, increased pulmonary vascular resistance leading to decrease in left to right shunt at PDA, is difficult to identify. Hemodynamic changes 20-30 min post administration may be the result of decreased venous return secondary to high PEEP and mean airway pressure. Pulmonary hemorrhage, and pneumothorax are less reported due lung protective strategies [55, 64-66].

Conclusion

Multitude of studies performed in adults, pediatrics and neonates have not yielded conclusive results due to limitations in effective surfactant delivery, phospholipase A2 inactivation of surfactant, surfactant injuring agents, lack of adequate dosing, and wrongful trial designs due to different preparations, patients and pathophysiology and comorbidities. Future studies should apply current definitions of PARDS and neonatal RDS in randomized trials evaluating efficacy of dose to dose between types of surfactants, routes of administration, in different patient population.

References

[1] Martin R. Pathophysiology, clinical manifestations, and diagnosis of respiratory distress syndrome in the newborn. In: Garcia-Prats JA WL, editor. *UpToDate.* Waltham, MA. (Accessed on June 05, 2022).

[2] Nkadi PO, Merritt TA, Pillers DA. An overview of pulmonary surfactant in the neonate: genetics, metabolism, and the role of surfactant in health and disease. *Mol Genet Metab.* 2009;97(2):95-101.

[3] Fessler MB, Summer RS. Surfactant Lipids at the Host-Environment Interface. Metabolic Sensors, Suppressors, and Effectors of Inflammatory Lung Disease. *Am J Respir Cell Mol Biol.* 2016;54(5):624-35.

[4] Whitsett JA, Wert SE, Weaver TE. Alveolar surfactant homeostasis and the pathogenesis of pulmonary disease. *Annu Rev Med.* 2010;61:105-19.

[5] Nogee L, Garnier G, Dietz H, Singer L, Murphy A, DeMello D, Coltent H. A Mutation in the Surfactant Protein B Gene Responsible for Fatal Neonatal Respiratory Disease in Multiple Kindreds. *Journal of Clinical Investigation.* 1994; 93(4):1860-3.

[6] Cochrane CR, SD. Pulmonary Surfactant Protein B (SP-B)- Structure-Function Relationships. *Science.* 1991;254:566-8.

[7] Nogee LM, Dunbar AE, Wert AE, Askin F, Hamvas A, Whitsett JA. A Mutation in The Surfactant Protein C Gene Associated with Familial Interstitial Lung Disease. *N Engl J Med.* 2001;344(8).

[8] Wu H, Kuzmenko A, Wan S, Schaffer L, Weiss A, Fisher JH, Sik Kim K, McCormack FX. Surfactant proteins A and D inhibit the growth of Gram-negative bacteria by increasing membrane permeability. *J Clin Invest.* 2003;111:1589-602.

[9] Sato A, Whitsett JA, Scheule RK, Ikegami M. Surfactant protein-d inhibits lung inflammation caused by ventilation in premature newborn lambs. *Am J Respir Crit Care Med.* 2010;181(10):1098-105.

[10] Ueda T Ikegami M, Jobe A. Surfactant subtypes. *In vitro* conversion, *in vivo* function, and effects of serum proteins. *Am J Respir Crit Care Med.* 1994;149(5).

[11] Rogulska J, Wroblewska-Seniuk K, Smigiel R, Szydlowski J, Szczapa T. Diagnostic Challenges in Neonatal Respiratory Distress-Congenital Surfactant Metabolism Dysfunction Caused by ABCA3 Mutation. *Diagnostics.* 2022;12(5).

[12] Townsel CD, Emmer SF, Campbell WA, Hussain N. Gender Differences in Respiratory Morbidity and Mortality of Preterm Neonates. *Front Pediatr.* 2017;5:6.

[13] Carlton DP AK, Cho SC, Lont M, Bland RD. Role of neutrophils in lung vascular injury and edema after premature birth in lambs. *J Appl Physiol.* 1997;83(4):1307.

[14] Nitta K, Kobayashi T. Impairment of surfactant activity and ventilation by proteins in lung edema fluid. *Respir Physiol.* 1994;95(1): 43.

[15] Bae CT, A. Chida, S. Sasaki, M. Morphology and Function of Pulmonary Surfactant Inhibited by Meconium. *Pediatric Research.* 1998;44:187-91.

[16] Schrama AJ, de Beaufort AJ, Sukul YR, Jansen SM, Poorthuis BJ, Berger HM. Phospholipase A2 is present in meconium and inhibits the activity of pulmonary surfactant *in vitro*. *Acta Pediatr.* 2001;90:412-6.

[17] Kaapa P, Soukka H. Phospholipase A2 in meconium-induced lung injury. *J Perinatol.* 2008;28 Suppl 3:S120-2.

[18] Haas NA, Kulasekaran K, Camphausen CK. Successful use of surfactant to treat severe intrapulmonary hemorrhage after iatrogenic lung injury--A case report. *Pediatr Crit Care Med.* 2006;7(6):583-5.

[19] Echaide M, Autilio C, Arroyo R, Perez-Gil J. Restoring pulmonary surfactant membranes and films at the respiratory surface. *Biochim Biophys Acta Biomembr.* 2017;1859(9 Pt B):1725-39.

[20] Yuan J, Chiofolo CM, Czerwin BJ, Karamolegkos N, Chbat NW. Alveolar Tissue Fiber and Surfactant Effects on Lung Mechanics-Model Development and Validation on ARDS and IPF Patients. *IEEE Open J Eng Med Biol* .2021;2:44-54.

[21] Pison UT, Tam EK, Caughey GH, Hawgood S. Proteolytic inactivation of dog lung surfactant-associated proteins by neutrophil elastase. *Biochimica et Biophysica Acta.* 1989;992(3):251-7.

[22] Baker CE, TW. Randle, BJ. Haslam, PL. Damage to surfactant-specific protein in acute respiratory distress syndrome. *The Lancet.* 1999;353(9160):1232-7.

[23] Lim M, Zinter M, Bhalla A, Orwoll B, Alkhouli M, Raitu A, Chen L, Gug-lielmo M, Gala K, Sapru A. Plasma Surfactant Protein-D Is an Early Prognostic Marker of Mortality Among Pediatric ARDS Patients. *Crit Care Med.* 2018;47(1):1223.

[24] Wolfler A, Piastra M, Amigoni A, Santuz P, Gitto E, Rossetti E, Tinelli C, Montani C, Savron F, Simone P, D'amato L, Mondardini MC, Conti G, De Silvestri A. A shared protocol for porcine surfactant use in pediatric acute respiratory distress syndrome: a feasibility study. *BMC Pediatr.* 2019;19(1):203.

[25] Deutsch GH, Young LR, Deterding RR, Fan LL, Dell SD, Bean JA, Brody AS, Nogee LM, Bruce CT, Langston C, and the Pathology Cooperative Group: Albright EA, Askin FB, Baker P, Chou PM, Cool CM, Coventry SC, Cutz E, Davis MM, Dishop MK, Galalbos C, Patterson K, Travis WD, Wert S, White FV, on behalf of the ChILD Research Co-operative. Diffuse lung disease in young children: application of a novel classification scheme. *Am J Respir Crit Care Med.* 2007; 176(11):1120-8.

[26] Suzuki T, Sakagami T, Young LR, Carey BC, Wood RE, Luisetti M, Wert SE, Rubin BK, Kevill K, Chalk C, Whitsett JA, Stevens C, Nogee LM, Campo I, Trapnell BC. Hereditary pulmonary alveolar proteinosis: pathogenesis, presentation, diagnosis, and therapy. *Am J Respir Crit Care Med.* 2010;182(10): 1292-304.

[27] Suzuki T, Sakagami T, Rubin BK, Nogee LM, Wood RE, Zimmerman SL, Smolarek T, Dishop MK, Wert SE, Whitsett JA, Grabowski G, Carey BC, Stevens C, van der Loo JCM, Trapnell C. Familial pulmonary alveolar proteinosis caused by mutations in CSF2RA. *J Exp Med.* 2008;205(12):2703-10.

[28] Nogee LG, WA. Genetic disorders of surfactant dysfunction. In: Mallory GH, AG., editor. *UpToDate,* Waltham, MA. (Accessed on June 08, 2022).

[29] Brasch F, Griese M, Tredano M, Johnen G, Ochs M, Rieger C, Mulugeta S, Muller KM, Bahuau M, Beers MF. Interstitial lung disease in a baby with a de novo mutation in the SFTPC gene. *Eur Respir J.* 2004;24(1):30-9.

[30] Shulenin S NL, Annilo T, Wert SE, Whitsett JA, Dean M. ABCA3 gene mutations in newborns with fatal surfactant deficiency. *N Engl J Med.* 2004;350(13):1296.

[31] Garmany TH, Wambach JA, Heins HB, Watkins-Torry JM, Wegner DJ, Bennet, K, An P, Land G, Saugstad OD, Henderson H, Nogee LM, Cole FS, Hamvas A. Population and Disease-Based Prevalence of the Common Mutations Associated with Surfactant Deficiency. *Pediatr Res.* 2008;63:645–9.

[32] Willson DF, Jiao JH, Bauman LA, Zaritsky A, Craft H, Dockery K, Conrad D, Dalton H. Calf lung surfactant extract in acute hypoxemic respiratory failure in children. *Crit Care Med.* 1996;24:1316–1322.

[33] Willson DF, Zaritsky A, Bauman LA, Dockery K, James RL, Conrad D, Craft H, Novotny WE, Egan EA, Dalton H. Instillation of calf lung surfactant extract (calfactant) is beneficial in pediatric acute hypoxemic respiratory failure. *Crit Care Med.* 1999; 27:188–195.

[34] Willson DF, Thomas NJ, Markovitz BP, Bauman LA, DiCarlo JV, Pon S, Jacobs BR, Jefferson LS, Conway MR, Egan EA. Effect of exogenous surfactant (calfactant) in pediatric acute lung injury: A randomized controlled trial. *JAMA.* 2005; 293:470–476.

[35] Gregory TJ, Steinberg KP, Spragg R, Gadek JE, Hyers TM, Longmore WJ, Moxley MA, Cai GZ, Hite RD, Smith RM, Hudson LD, Crim C, Newton P, Mitchell BR, Gold AJ. Bovine surfactant therapy for patients with acute respiratory distress syndrome. *Am J Respir Crit Care Med.* 1997;155:1309–1315.

[36] Tridente A, De Martino L, De Luca D. Porcine vs bovine surfactant therapy for preterm neonates with RDS: systematic review with biological plausibility and pragmatic meta-analysis of respiratory outcomes. *Respiratory Research.* 2019;20: 28.

[37] Hentschel R, Bohlin K, van Kaam A, Fuchs H, Danhaive O. Surfactant replacement therapy: from biological basis to current clinical practice. *Pediatric Research.* 2020;88:176-183.

[38] Ramanathan R, Bhatia JJ, Sekar K, Ernst FR. Mortality in preterm infants with respiratory distress syndrome treated with poractant alfa, calfactant or beractant: retrospective study. *J Perinatol.* 2013 Feb; 33(2):119-25.

[39] Singh N, Halliday HL, Stevens TP, Suresh G, Soll R, Rojas- Reyes MX. Comparison of animal-derived surfactants for the prevention and treatment of respiratory distress syndrome in preterm infants. *Cochrane Database Syst Rev.* 2015 Dec 21; (12):CD010249.

[40] Sinha SK, Lacaze-Masmonteil T, Valls I Soler A, Wiswell TE, Gadzinowski J, Hajdu J, Bernstein G, Sanchez-Luna M, Segal R, Schaber CJ, Massaro J, d Agostino R, Surfaxin Therapy Against Respiratory Distress Syndrome Collaborative Group. A multicenter, randomized, controlled trial of lucinanctant versus poractant alfa among very premature infants at high risk for respiratory distress syndrome. *Pediatrics.* 2005;115(4):1030-8.

[41] Moya FR, Gadzinowski J, Bancalari E, Salinas V, Kopelman B, Bancalari A, Kornacka MK, Meritt TA, Segal R, Schaber CJ, Tsai H, Massaro J, d'Agostino R, international surfaxin collaborative study group. A multicenter, randomized, masked, comparision trial of lucinactant, colfosceril palmitate, and beractant for the

prevention of respiratory distress syndrome among very preterm infants. *Pediatrics.* 2005;115(4):1018-29.

[42] Spragg RG, Lewis JF, Walmrath HD, Johnnigman J, Bellingan G, Laterre PF, Witte MC, Richards GA, Rippin G, Rathgeb F, Hafner D, Taut JH, Seeger W. Effect of Recombinant Surfactant Protein C – Based Surfactant on the Acute Respiratory Distress Syndrome. *N Engl J Med.* 2004;351:884-92.

[43] Moller JC, Schaible T, Roll C, Schiffmann JH, Bindl L, Schrod L, Reiss I, Kohl M, Demirakca S, Hentschel R, Paul T, Vierzig A, Groneck P, von Seefeld H, Schumacher H, Gortner L, Surfactant ARDS study group. Treatment with bovine surfactant in severe acute respiratory distress syndrome in children: a randomized multicenter study. *Intensive Care Med.* 2003;29:437-446.

[44] Lotze A, Knight GR, Martin GR, Bulas DI, Hull WM, O'Donnell RM, Whitsett JA, Short BL. Improved pulmonary outcome after exogenous surfactant therapy. *J Pediatr.* 1993; 122(2):261-8.

[45] Thomas NJ, Spear D, Wasserman E, Pon S, Markovitz B, Singh AR, Li S, Gertz SJ, Rowan CM, Kunselman A, Tamburro RF. CALIPSO: A Randomized Controlled Trial of Calfactant for Acute Lung Injury in Pediatric Stem cell and Oncology Patients. *Biol Blood marrow Transplant.* 2018; 24(12):2479-2486.

[46] Willson DF, Thomas NJ, Tamburro R, Truemper E, Truwit J, Conaway M, Traul C, Egan EE, Pediatric Acute Lung and Sepsis Investigators Network. Pediatric Calfactant in acute respiratory distress syndrome trial. *Pediatr Crit Care Med.* 2013;14:657-665.

[47] Thomas NJ, Guardia CG, Moya FR, Cheifetz I, Markovitz B, Cruces P, Barton P, Segal R, Simmons P, Randolph AG, PALISI Network. A pilot randomized controlled clinical trial of Lucinactant, a peptide-containing synthetic surfactant, in infants with acute hypoxemic respiratory failure. *Pediatr Crit Care Med.* 2012;13 (6):646-53.

[48] Raghavendran K, Wilson D, Notter RH. Surfactant Therapy of ALI and ARDS. *Crit Care Clin.* 2011; 27(3):525-559.

[49] Findlay RD, Taeusch HW, Walther FJ. Surfactant replacement therapy for meconium aspiration syndrome. *Pediatrics.* 1996;97(11):48-52.

[50] El Shahed AI, Dargaville PA, Ohlsson A, Soll R. Surfactant for meconium aspiration syndrome in term and late preterm infants. *Cochrane Database Syst Rev.* 2014;(12):CD002054.

[51] Polin RA, Carlo WA, Committee on Fetus and Newborn; American Academy of Pediatrics. Surfactant Replacement Therapy for preterm and term infants Neonates with Respiratory Distress. Clinical Report. *Pediatrics.* 2014;133(1):156-163.

[52] Minocchieri S, Berry CA, Pillow JJ, Cure Neb Study Team. Nebulised surfactant to reduce severity of respiratory distress: a blinded, parallel, randomized controlled trial. *Arch Dis Child Fetal Neonatal Ed.* 2019;104(3):F313-F319.

[53] Berggren E, Liljedahl M, Windladh B, Andreasson B, Curstedt T, Robertson B, Schollin J. Pilot study of nebulized surfactant therapy for neonatal respiratory distress syndrome. *Acta Paediatr.* 2000;89(4):460-4.

[54] Schermuky RT, Gunther A, Weissmann N, Ghofrani HA, Seeger W, Grimminger F, Walmrath D. Differential Impact of ultrasonically nebulized versus Tracheal

instilled surfactant on ventilation-Perfusion (Va/Q) mismatch in a model of acute lung injury. *Am J Respir Crit Care Med.* 2000;161:152-159.

[55] Shein SL, Maul TM, Li H, Kurland G. Surfactant Administration During Pediatric Extracorporeal Membrane Oxygenation. *ASAIO J.* 2015;61(6):682-7.

[56] Chrysostomou C, Maul T, Istvanic F, Wearden P. Surfactant Administration During Pediatric Cardiac Extracorporeal Membrane Oxygenation. *ASAIO J.* 2019;65(4): 367-370.

[57] Hermon M, Burda G, Male C, Boigner H, Ponhold W, Khoss A, Strohmaier W, Trittenwein G. Surfactant application during extracorporeal membrane oxygenation improves lung volume and pulmonary mechanics in children with respiratory failure. *Critical Care.* 2005;9(6):R718-24.

[58] Qaqish R, Watanabe Y, Galasso M, Summers C, Ali A, Takahashi M, Gazzalle A, Liu M, Keshavjee S, Cypel M, Del Sorbo L. Veno-venous ECMO as a platform to evaluate lung lavage and surfactant replacement therapy in an animal model of severe ARDS. *Intensive Care Med Exp.* 2020;8(1):63.

[59] Crouch E, Wright JR. Surfactant Proteins A and D and Pulmonary Host Defense. *Annu Rev Physiol.* 2001;63:521-54.

[60] Foo SS, Reading PC, Jallion S, Mantovani A, Mahalingam S. Pentraxins and Collectins: Friend or Foe during Pathogen Invasion?. *Trends Microbiol.* 2015; 23(12):799-811.

[61] Dahl M, Holmskov U, Husby S, Juvonen PO. Surfactant Protein D Levels in Umbilical Cord Blood and Capillary Blood of Premature Infants. The Influence of Perinatal Factors. *Pediatric Research.* 2006;59:806-810.

[62] Dhmer MK, Flori H, Sapru A, Kohne J, Weeks HM, Curley MAQ, Matthay MA, Quasney MW. Surfactant protein D Is Associated With Severe Pediatric ARDS, Prolonged Ventilation, and Death in Children With Acute Respiratory Failure. *Chest.* 2020;158(3):1027-1035.

[63] Orwoll BE, Sapru A. Biomarkers in Pediatric ARDS: Future Directions. *Front. Pediatr.* 2016;4:55.

[64] Schmolzer GM, Kamlin COF, Dawson JA, Morley CJ, Davis PG. Tidal volume delivery during surfactant administration in the delivery room. *Intensive Care Med.* 2011;37(11):1833-9.

[65] Hentschel R, Jorch G. Acute Side effects of Surfactant treatment. *J Perinat Med.* 2002;30(2):143-8.

[66] Long W, Corbet A, Cotton R, Courtney S, McGuiness G, Walter D, JWatts J, Smyth J, Bard H, Chernick V, the American Exosurf Neonatal Study Group I, and the Canadian Exosurf Neonatal Study Group. A controlled trial of synthetic surfactant in infants weighing 1250 g or more with respiratory distress syndrome. *N Engl J Med.* 1991;325:1696-1703.

Chapter 18

Lung-Protective Ventilation Strategies in Preterm Infants

M. O'Reilly[1,2], PhD
and G. M. Schmölzer[1,2,*], MD, PhD
[1] Centre for the Studies of Asphyxia and Resuscitation,
Neonatal Research Unit, Royal Alexandra Hospital, Edmonton, Alberta, Canada
[2] Department of Pediatrics, University of Alberta, Edmonton, Alberta, Canada

Abstract

Around 10-20% of newborns (approximately 13-26 million worldwide) require non-invasive or invasive respiratory support from birth. Extremely preterm infants have difficulties in establishing effective breathing after birth as their lungs are structurally immature, surfactant-deficient, and not supported by a stiff chest wall. Preterm infants are vulnerable to ventilator-induced lung injury (VILI) because their partially fluid-filled immature lungs, which are not uniformly ventilated and often surfactant-deficient.

The use of ventilation strategies in the delivery room and in the neonatal intensive care unit to establish a functional residual capacity and maintain lung aeration and oxygenation, although lifesaving in many cases, can also injure the lung and cause various traumas at a cellular level. Mechanical ventilation can injure the preterm lungs and multiple ventilation strategies have been postulated to reduce VILI and improve outcomes.

---

* Corresponding Author's Email: georg.schmoelzer@me.com.

In: Ventilator Induced Lung Injury in Non-Invasive Ventilatory Support
Editor: Antonio M. Esquinas
ISBN: 979-8-88697-840-7

Keywords: lung injury, preterm infants, delivery room, neonatal intensive care unit, mechanical ventilation

Introduction

When newborn infants fail to initiate spontaneous breathing [1], various evidence-based international and national resuscitation guidelines recommend equipment and techniques for neonatal resuscitation [2–4]. These guidelines all agree that positive pressure ventilation (PPV) is the cornerstone of respiratory support immediately after birth [5]. Current neonatal resuscitation guidelines recommend initiation of PPV if the heart rate is < 100 beats per minute [2, 3].

The purpose of PPV is to create a functional residual capacity in the lungs, deliver an adequate tidal volume (V_T), facilitate gas exchange, and stimulate breathing, all while minimizing lung injury [5]. In the delivery room, PPV is routinely provided via a face mask connected to a pressure-limited device (called a T-piece resuscitator), and a peak inflation pressure (PIP) is somewhat arbitrarily chosen, with the assumption an adequate V_T will be delivered [2, 3]. However, the delivered V_T is rarely measured and therefore PIP is not adjusted to optimize V_T delivery [2, 3].

Reduction of Lung Injury during Neonatal Resuscitation in the Delivery Room

Continuous Positive Airway Pressure

Observational studies reported lower rates of bronchopulmonary dysplasia in centers who used nasal continuous positive airway pressure (CPAP) shortly after birth [6-8]. A further observational study reported rates of bronchopulmonary dysplasia in two Boston centres (22%) with a single centre in New York (4%), which was related to increased use of mechanical ventilation (Boston 75% vs New York 29%) [9]. These observational studies suggest that high delivery room intubation rates are associated with higher rates of bronchopulmonary dysplasia.

This led to large randomised controlled trials comparing primary nasal CPAP with endotracheal intubation and mechanical ventilation after birth for the prevention of death or bronchopulmonary dysplasia in very preterm infants [10-12]. A total of four trials including 2,782 (nasal CPAP n = 1,296 and intubation n = 1,486) infants were included in a meta-analysis [13]. The relative risk (95% confidence interval (CI)) of bronchopulmonary dysplasia was 0.91, (0.82 to 1.01), risk difference (95%CI) −0.03 (−0.07 to 0.01), of death relative risk (95% CI) 0.88 (0.68 to 1.14), risk difference (95%CI) −0.02 (−0.04 to 0.01).

While neither bronchopulmonary dysplasia or death was significantly reduced, the pooled analysis revealed a significant benefit for the combined outcome of death or bronchopulmonary dysplasia, or both for babies treated with nasal CPAP relative risk (95% CI) 0.91 (0.84 to 0.99), risk difference (95% CI) −0.04 (-0.07 to 0.00). This suggests that for every 25 infants treated with CPAP instead of intubation and mechanical ventilation after birth, one additional infant could survive to 36 weeks without bronchopulmonary dysplasia [13].

Positive Pressure Ventilation

It is imperative that a lung-protective strategy starts immediately after birth [5]. The volume difference between functional residual capacity and total lung capacity is small in very preterm newborns [14]. Lung compliance and the corresponding PIP needed to deliver an appropriate V_T vary greatly in the first minutes after birth [15], and depend on the prematurity of the newborn, disease state, delivery mode (C-section vs. vaginal birth), and degree of lung aeration [15]. Therefore, relying on a fixed PIP may result in harm by either under- or over-inflating the lung [5]. It is therefore necessary to measure and adjust the V_T delivered during PPV in the minutes after birth, especially in preterm infants at the greatest risk of lung injury [16, 17].

Using a face mask to deliver PPV can often lead to large and variable gas leak between the mask and face [16, 18–24]. Indeed, delivery room studies reported that mask leak varies widely during PPV [median (range) mask leak of 29% (0-100%)], with most resuscitators being unaware of the extent of their mask leak [23, 24]. Face mask leak occurs frequently, even for experienced resuscitators, and seriously affects the delivered V_T [25]. The V_T changes as the leak changes, even though the same PIP is used. In practice, this means that for the same PIP the V_T may be low, appropriate, or [26] excessive depending on mask leak.

Delivery room studies have reported that the delivered V_T during mask PPV ranges between 0-31 mL/kg [23, 27–30]. This is concerning because animal studies have demonstrated that lung injury is predominantly caused by high V_T ventilation (> 8 mL/kg) and not by high pressure per se [31, 32].

A respiratory function monitor (RFM), which displays delivered pressures and volumes, has been postulated to reduce mask leak [21], thus improving the delivered V_T and effectiveness of PPV. Simulated training studies in mannequins demonstrated that mask leak was reduced when resuscitators were able to view the RFM and receive immediate visual and numerical feedback [33]. Randomized trials in the delivery room reported that utilizing an RFM during PPV allows the resuscitator to target V_T and is associated with a lower rate of excessive (> 8 mL/kg) V_T delivery. Schmölzer et al., compared V_T delivery with an RFM visible vs. clinical assessment (RFM masked) during mask PPV in the delivery room in preterm infants < 32 weeks' gestation and reported similar V_T in both groups (5.7 mL/kg in the RFM visible group vs. 5.6 mL/kg in the RFM masked group) [28]. However, both the proportion of infants with a V_T > 8 mL/kg (0.81; 95% CI, 0.67-0.98) and the mean/median mask leak was a significantly lower when the RFM was visible (37% vs. 54%, $p = 0.01$) [28].

In comparison, Zeballos et al., reported significantly lower V_T in the RFM visible vs. no RFM group with 5.8 (4.7–6.8) and 7 (5.7– 9.2) mL/kg ($p < 0.001$), respectively [30]. van Zanten et al., reported no difference in median (IQR) V_T between the RFM group and no RFM group [5.1 (4-7.1) and 5.9 (4.2-8.4) mL/kg, $p = 0.057$] [29]. Overall, these three trials confirm that the proportion of infants receiving V_T > 8 mL/kg can be reduced with an RFM visible. Although an RFM during PPV in the delivery room reduced the proportion of inflations with a V_T > 8 mL/kg, a high V_T (> 8 mL/kg) was still delivered in ~30% of inflations. Furthermore, rates of mortality or bronchopulmonary dysplasia were unchanged in all trials [34]. This indicates that an RFM to adjust V_T may not be the optimal approach. Therefore, alternate methods of providing tight V_T control during PPV in the delivery room resuscitation of preterm infants is needed, given the complex interaction of mask leak, lung compliance, PIP, and resuscitator skill.

Volume-controlled ventilation in the delivery room, rather than pressure-driven resuscitation, may enhance lung protection in the first moments following birth. Volume-targeted ventilation devices have been assessed during simulated neonatal resuscitation in mannequins [35, 36]. In two simulation studies, Solevåg et al., assessed mask ventilation using a volume-controlled prototype device and compared it to standard pressure devices, including the self-inflating bag and various T-piece resuscitators [35, 36]. In a high airway compliance mannequin test lung, V_T delivery was two-fold to six-fold higher than the target V_T when standard resuscitation devices were used [35, 36]. In contrast, the volume-controlled prototype device delivered a lower V_T during mask ventilation and was shown to have the most consistent V_T delivery and ventilation rate compared to the other standard devices [35, 36].

Other simulation studies have also investigated volume-controlled resuscitation strategies. Tracy et al., compared mask PPV with a T-Piece or volume-targeted ventilator during simulated neonatal resuscitation and reported a lower coefficient of variations and lower V_T delivery with ventilator driven volume-targeted ventilation compared to PPV with a T-piece [37]. Similarly, Jain et al., compared volume-targeted ventilation via a mechanical ventilator to manual T-piece PPV and reported improved volume targeting at different compliance settings and a reduction in mask leak during simulated mask ventilation [38]. These simulated studies indicate that volume-targeted neonatal resuscitation has the potential to provide a lung-protective strategy from birth, however further investigation and clinical trials are warranted.

Strategies to Reduce Lung Injury during Respiratory Support in NICU

Neonatologists are increasingly careful in the NICU to apply ventilation strategies that are gentle to the lungs [39–43]. The function of mechanical ventilation is to ventilate and oxygenate the lung via a constant end-expiratory pressure and intermittent inflation pressures either using a flow- or time-cycled approach with an inflation rate which mimics physiologic breathing rates of newborn infants. To achieve this gas is pumped mechanically into the lungs using either a set pressure or set tidal volume. The delivered tidal volume will depend on the lung disease stage and disease origin which can result in reduced compliance, high resistance, and/or air trapping. These circumstances often result in insufficient inspiratory or expiratory time to allow the lung to oxygenate and ventilate sufficiently.

During mechanical ventilation, the lung should be divided into several zones: At any given time, the lung could be divided into a healthy, a recruitable, and a diseased lung unresponsive to pressure changes. Alternatively, the lung could be divided into an aerated, hyper-inflated, and an under-inflated or atelectatic lung. Further, the difference in volume between functional residual capacity and total lung capacity is small in preterm infants [44, 45]. In term infants, the total lung capacity is between 43 to 52 mL/kg [14] while preterm infants with respiratory distress syndrome have a functional residual capacity of ~11 mL/kg and a total lung capacity of ~19 ml/kg [14].

This suggests that mechanical ventilation with combinations of functional residual capacities and tidal volumes who in sum exceeds total lung capacity that rather just a tidal volume of greater than 8 mL/kg would result in lung damage. This is further supported by tidal volume measurements in spontaneously breathing preterm infants born < 32 weeks' gestations which ranges between 3 to 7.5 mL/kg) [46–49]. To minimize lung injury during mechanical ventilation, clinicians might consider tidal volumes targets which are most used in the NICU of 4 to 6 mL/kg may be a good starting point [43].

Non-Invasive Ventilation

Continuous Positive Airway Pressure

Although, several large, randomized trials and meta-analysis comparing CPAP to intubation and mechanical ventilation in the delivery room reported only a minor effect on chronic lung disease [50], the available evidence supports CPAP to reduce the need for mechanical ventilation and chronic lung disease [51]. There are several different approaches to provide CPAP including bubble CPAP, bilevel CPAP, bilevel positive airway pressure, or nasal intermittent positive-pressure ventilation (NIPPV).

In animal studies, bubble CPAP improve gas exchange and decreased markers of lung injury, which might be due to the oscillatory effect. A recent meta-analysis reported a reduced incidence of CPAP failure with bubble CPAP compared to ventilator CPAP.

Bilevel CPAP, which cycles between two set pressure levels, does not allow comparing for synchronization with spontaneous breathing nor produces a measurable tidal volume, which did not improve outcomes [52, 53].

NIPPV is a further non-invasive respiratory support modality, which is most commonly used to reduce post-extubation failure [54]. Although reducing post-extubation failure is desired by neonatologists to reduce the VILI (potential effects of invasive ventilation), the effects of lower reintubation rates is mainly driven by using higher MAP with NIPPV compared with CPAP [51]. Therefore, studies comparing similar mean airway pressures using both CPAP and NIPPV (ClinicalTrials.gov Identifier NCT03512158 and NCT03670732) are currently underway.

Volume-Targeted Ventilation

Volume-targeted ventilation (VTV), where ventilators algorithmically adjust the PIP to target a set tidal volume, as detected through an inline flow sensor, is routinely used in the NICU [40, 42, 43]. Meta-analysis comparing pressure-targeted with volume-targeted ventilation in the NICU reported a reduction in a number of adverse clinical endpoints [42, 55], including, 1) the incidence of pneumothorax (typical RR [95%CI] 0.46 [0.25-0.84], numbers needed to treat [95%CI] 17 [10-100]), 2) hypocarbia (typical RR [95%CI] 0.56 [0.33-0.96], numbers needed to treat [95%CI] 4 [2-25]), 3) combined outcome of death or bronchopulmonary dysplasia (typical RR [95%CI] 0.73 [0.57-0.93], numbers needed to treat [95%CI] 8 [5-33]), and iv) the combined outcome of periventricular leukomalacia (PVL) or grade 3-4 IVH (typical RR [95%CI] 0.48 [0.28-0.84], numbers needed to treat [95%CI] 11 [7-50]).

High Frequency Oscillatory Ventilation

An alternative approach to mechanical ventilation is high frequency oscillatory ventilation (HFOV), which is most used as a rescue mode, when clinicians struggle to oxygenate and/or ventilate a newborn infant [43]. HFOV uses a constant mean airway pressure around which a diaphragm oscillates at a set amplitude resulting in active inspiration and expiration.

There are multiple theoretical mechanisms on how ventilation and/or gas exchange occurs during HFOV including:

1) Direct alveolar ventilation of lung units near airway opening.
2) Pendelluft, which describes the bulk convective mixing in conducting airways as a result of recirculation of air between units of inhomogeneous time constants.
3) Convective gas transport as a result of asymmetry between inspiratory and expiratory velocity profiles.
4) Longitudinal dispersion due to interaction between axial velocities and radial transports (Taylor-type dispersion).
5) Molecular diffusion near the alveolocapillary membrane [51].

There is limited evidence for HFOV in as initial treatment for infants with uncomplicated respiratory distress syndrome. Early on, HFOV has been used more like a “rescue ventilation approach” in infants on conventional mechanical ventilation with severe respiratory failure due to ventilation or oxygenation failures. Randomized trials and meta-analyses comparing conventional mechanical ventilation with HFOV in premature infants with respiratory distress reported similar incidence of chronic lung disease and mortality when HFOV as a rescue mode was used. More recently, HFOV has been used more electively as a first line treatment option in respiratory distress, which has been associated with a potential reduction in chronic lung disease. Currently HFOV is used for congenital diaphragmatic hernia, meconium aspiration syndrome, respiratory distress syndrome, persistent pulmonary hypertension, pulmonary hypoplasia, and chronic lung disease [51].

A novel ventilation mode within HFOV, is the possibility to combine volume guarantee (VG) with HFOV (= HFOV + VG), which uses a similar approach as VTV in conventional mechanical ventilation. HFOV + VG might reduce inadvertent overventilation that occurs during HFOV and thereby effect CO_2 elimination and ventilation efficiency [51]. A multicenter trial (ClinicalTrials.gov Identifier NCT02445040) has recently been completed and results are awaited.

Automated Control of Fraction of Inspired Oxygen

Automated control of oxygen delivery has recently gained interest to:

1) Reduce the percent of time infants spend outside target oxygen saturation.
2) Severe oxygen saturation deviations.
3) Need for manual oxygen adjustments [51, 56, 57].

This technology allows to reduce hyperoxemia and hypoxemia and thereby reduce oxidative stress and pro-inflammatory stimuli with the potential to reduce the risk of bronchopulmonary dysplasia.

Conclusion

Lung protective ventilation strategies for extremely preterm infant should start immediately after birth and will requires knowledge of the respiratory pathophysiology and a ventilation strategy to recruit the lung while not over distending or collapsing the lung.

References

[1] Aziz K, Chadwick M, Baker M, Andrews W. Ante- and intra-partum factors that predict increased need for neonatal resuscitation. *Resuscitation*. 2008 Dec;79(3): 444–52.

[2] Aziz K, Lee H C, Escobedo M B, Hoover A V, Kamath-Rayne B D, Kapadia V S, Magid D J, Niermeyer S, Schmölzer G M, Szyld E G, Weiner G M, Wyckoff M H, Yamada N K, Zaichkin J. Part 5: Neonatal Resuscitation: 2020 American Heart Association Guidelines for Cardiopulmonary Resuscitation and Emergency Cardiovascular Care. *Circulation*. 2020 Oct 20;142(16_suppl_2):1–27.

[3] Wyckoff M H, Wyllie J P, Aziz K, Almeida M F de, Fabres J, Fawke J, et al. Neonatal Life Support: 2020 International Consensus on Cardiopulmonary Resuscitation and Emergency Cardiovascular Care Science With Treatment Recommendations. *Circulation*. 2020 Oct 20;142(16_suppl_1):329–37.

[4] Madar J, Roehr C C, Ainsworth S, Ersdal H, Morley C, Rüdiger M, Skåre C, Szczapa T, Pas A te, Trevisanuto D, Urlesberger B, Wilkinson D, Wyllie J P. European Resuscitation Council Guidelines 2021: Newborn resuscitation and support of transition of infants at birth. *Resuscitation*. 2021;161:291–326.

[5] Schmölzer G M, te Pas A B, Davis P G, Morley C J. Reducing lung injury during neonatal resuscitation of preterm infants. *J. Pediatr*. 2008 Dec;153(6):741–5.

[6] Avery M E, Tooley W H, Keller J B, Hurd S S, Bryan M H, Cotton R B, Epstein M F, Fitzhardinge P M, Hansen C B, Hansen T N, Hodson W A, James L S, Kitterman J A, Nielsen H C, Poirier T A, Truog W E, Wung J T. Is chronic lung disease in low birth weight infants preventable? A survey of eight centers. *Pediatrics* 1987;79:26-30.

[7] Van Marter L J, Allred E N, Pagano M, Sanocka U, Parad R, Moore M, Susser M, Paneth N, Leviton A. Do clinical markers of barotrauma and oxygen toxicity explain interhospital variation in rates of chronic lung disease? The Neonatology Committee for the Developmental Network. *Pediatrics* 2000;105:1194-201.

[8] Ammari A, Suri M, Milisavljevic V, Sahni R, Bateman D, Sanocka U, Ruzal-Shapiro C, Wung J T, Polin R A. Variables associated with the early failure of nasal CPAP in very low birth weight infants. *J. Pediatr*. 2005;147:341-7.

[9] Gagliardi L, Bellù R, Lista G, Zanini R, Network Neonatale Lombardo Study Group. Do differences in delivery room intubation explain different rates of bronchopulmonary dysplasia between hospitals? *Arch. Dis. Child. - Fetal Neonatal Ed.* 2011;96:F30-5.

[10] Morley C J, Davis P G, Doyle L W, Brion L P, Hascoet J M, Carlin J B, COIN Trial Investigators. Nasal CPAP or intubation at birth for very preterm infants. *N. Engl. J. Med.* 2008;358:700-8.

[11] SUPPORT Study Group of the Eunice Kennedy Shriver NICHD Neonatal Research Network, Finer N N, Carlo W A, Walsh M C, Rich W, Gantz M G, et al. Early CPAP versus surfactant in extremely preterm infants. *N. Engl. J. Med.* 2010;362:1970-9.

[12] Dunn M S, Kaempf J, de Klerk A, de Klerk R, Reilly M, Howard D, Ferrelli K, O'Conor J, Soll R F, Vermont Oxford Network DRM Study Group. Randomized

trial comparing 3 approaches to the initial respiratory management of preterm neonates. *Pediatrics* 2011;128:e1069-76.

[13] Schmölzer G M, Kumar M, Pichler G, Aziz K, O'Reilly M, Cheung P Y. Non-invasive versus invasive respiratory support in preterm infants at birth: systematic review and meta-analysis. *BMJ* 2013 Oct 17;347:f5980. doi: 10.1136/bmj.f5980.

[14] Vilstrup C T, Björklund L J, Werner O, Larsson A. Lung Volumes and Pressure-Volume Relations of the Respiratory System in Small Ventilated Neonates with Severe Respiratory Distress Syndrome. *Pediatric Research*. 1996 Jan;39(1):127–33.

[15] te Pas A B, Davis P G, Hooper S B, Morley C J. From liquid to air: breathing after birth. *J. Pediatr*. 2008 May;152(5):607–11.

[16] Schmölzer G M, Kamlin C O F, Dawson J A, Pas A B te, Morley C J, Davis P G. Respiratory monitoring of neonatal resuscitation. *Archives of Disease in Childhood-Fetal and Neonatal Edition*. 2010 Jul;95(4):F295-303.

[17] Hooper S B, Fouras A, Siew M L, Wallace M J, Kitchen M, Pas AB te, Klingenberg C, Lewis R A, Davis P G, Morley C J, Schmölzer G M. Expired CO2 levels indicate degree of lung aeration at birth. *PLOS ONE*. 2013;8(8):e70895.

[18] Wood F E, Morley C J, Davis P G. A respiratory function monitor improves mask ventilation. *Archives of Disease in Childhood-Fetal and Neonatal Edition*. 2008 Sep;93(5):F380-1.

[19] Wood F E, Morley C J, Kamlin C O F, Owen L, Donath S, Davis P G. Assessing the effectiveness of two round neonatal resuscitation masks: study 1. *Archives of Disease in Childhood-Fetal and Neonatal Edition*. 2008 May 1;93(3):F235–7.

[20] Wood F E, Morley C J. Face mask ventilation--the dos and don'ts. *Seminars in Fetal and Neonatal Medicine*. 2013 Dec;18(6):344–51.

[21] Schilleman K, Witlox R S G M, Lopriore E, te Pas A B. Leak and obstruction with mask ventilation during simulated neonatal resuscitation. *Archives of Disease in Childhood-Fetal and Neonatal Edition*. 2010 Nov;95(6):F398-402.

[22] Kaufman J, Schmölzer G M, Kamlin C O F, Davis P G. Mask ventilation of preterm infants in the delivery room. *Archives of Disease in Childhood-Fetal and Neonatal Edition*. 2013 Sep;98(5):F405-10.

[23] Schmölzer G M, Kamlin O C O F, O'Donnell C P F, Dawson J A, Morley C J, Davis P G. Assessment of tidal volume and gas leak during mask ventilation of preterm infants in the delivery room. *Archives Dis. Child. - Fetal Neonatal. Ed.* 2010 Nov;95 (6):F393.

[24] Schmölzer G M, Dawson J A, Kamlin C O F, O'Donnell C P, Morley C J, Davis P G. Airway obstruction and gas leak during mask ventilation of preterm infants in the delivery room. *Archives Dis. Child. - Fetal Neonatal. Ed.* 2011 Jul;96(4):F254.

[25] O'Donnell C P F, Kamlin C O F, Davis P G, Morley C J. Neonatal resuscitation 1: a model to measure inspired and expired tidal volumes and assess leakage at the face mask. *Archives Dis. Child. - Fetal Neonatal. Ed.* 2005 Sep 1;90(5):F388.

[26] Björklund L J, Ingimarsson J, Curstedt T, John J, Robertson B, Werner O, Vilstrup C T. Manual Ventilation with a Few Large Breaths at Birth Compromises the Therapeutic Effect of Subsequent Surfactant Replacement in Immature Lambs. *Pediatric Research*. 1997 Sep;42(3):348–55.

[27] Dawson J A, Schmölzer G M, Kamlin C O F, te Pas A B, O'Donnell C P F, Donath S M, Davis P G, Morley C J. Oxygenation with T-Piece versus Self-Inflating Bag for Ventilation of Extremely Preterm Infants at Birth: A Randomized Controlled Trial. *J. Pediatrics.* 2011 Jun;158(6):912-918.e2.

[28] Schmölzer G M, Wong C, Dawson J A, Kamlin C O F, Donath S, Hooper S B, Davis P G. Respiratory function monitor guidance of mask ventilation in the delivery room: a feasibility study. *J. Pediatr.* 2012 Mar;160(3):377-381.e2.

[29] van Zanten H A, Kuypers K L A M, Zwet E W van, Vonderen J J van, Kamlin C O F, Springer L, Lista G, Cavigioli F, Vento M, Núñez-Ramiro A, Oberthuer A, Kribs A, Kuester H, Horn S, Weinberg D D, Foglia E E, Morley C J, Davis P G, te Pas A B. A multi-centre randomised controlled trial of respiratory function monitoring during stabilisation of very preterm infants at birth. *Resuscitation.* 2021; Oct:167: 137-325.

[30] Zeballos Sarrato G, Sánchez Luna M, Zeballos Sarrato S, Pérez Pérez A, Pescador Chamorro I, Bellón Cano J M. New Strategies of Pulmonary Protection of Preterm Infants in the Delivery Room with the Respiratory Function Monitoring. *American Journal of Perinatology*. 2019 Jan 8;(EFirst):1–9.

[31] Hernandez L A, Peevy K J, Moise A A, Parker J C. Chest wall restriction limits high airway pressure-induced lung injury in young rabbits. *Journal of Applied Physiology*. 1989 Jan 1;66(5):2364–8.

[32] Dreyfuss D, Saumon G. Barotrauma is volutrauma, but which volume is the one responsible? *Intens Care Med*. 1992;18(3):139–41.

[33] O'Currain E, Thio M, Dawson J A, Donath S, Davis P G. Respiratory monitors to teach newborn facemask ventilation: a randomised trial. *Archives of Disease in Childhood-Fetal and Neonatal Edition*. 2019 Jan 13;

[34] de Medeiros S M, Mangat A, Polglase G R, Sarrato G Z, Davis P G, Schmölzer G M. Respiratory function monitoring to improve the outcomes following neonatal resuscitation: a systematic review and meta-analysis. *Archives Dis. Child. - Fetal Neonatal Ed* 2022:fetalneonatal-2021-323017. https://doi.org/10.1136/archdischild-2021-323017.

[35] Solevåg A, Haemmerle E, van Os S, Bach K P, Cheung P Y, Schmölzer G M. A Novel Prototype Neonatal Resuscitator That Controls Tidal Volume and Ventilation Rate: A Comparative Study of Mask Ventilation in a Newborn Manikin. *Frontiers in Pediatrics*. 2016;4:129.

[36] Solevåg A, Haemmerle E, van Os S, Bach K P, Cheung P Y, Schmölzer G M. Comparison of positive pressure ventilation devices in a newborn manikin. *Journal of Maternal-Fetal and Neonatal Medicine*. 2017 Mar;30(5):595–9.

[37] Tracy M B, Klimek J, Coughtrey H, Shingde V, Ponnampalam G, Hinder M, Maheshwari R, Tracy S K. Ventilator-delivered mask ventilation compared with three standard methods of mask ventilation in a manikin model. *Archives of Disease in Childhood-Fetal and Neonatal Edition*. 2011 Apr 12;96(3):F201–5.

[38] Jain D, D'Ugard C, Aguilar A, Moral T del, Bancalari E, Claure N. Use of a Mechanical Ventilator with Respiratory Function Monitoring Provides More Consistent Ventilation during Simulated Neonatal Resuscitation. *Neonatology*. 2020;117(2):151–8.

[39] Wheeler K, Davis P G, Kamlin C O F, Morley C J. Assist control volume guarantee ventilation during surfactant administration. *Archives of Disease in Childhood-Fetal and Neonatal Edition*. 2009 Aug 21;94(5):F336–8.

[40] Klingenberg C, Wheeler K, Davis P G, Morley C J. A practical guide to neonatal volume guarantee ventilation. *Journal of Perinatology*. 2011 Jul 14;31(9):575–85.

[41] Wheeler K, Klingenberg C, Morley C J, Davis P G. Volume-Targeted versus Pressure-Limited Ventilation for Preterm Infants: A Systematic Review and Meta-Analysis. *Neonatology*. 2011;100(3):219–27.

[42] Klingenberg C, Wheeler K I, McCallion N, Morley C J, Davis P G. Volume-targeted versus pressure-limited ventilation in neonates. *Cochrane Db. Syst. Rev*. 2017;2017 (10):CD003666.

[43] van Kaam A H, Rimensberger P C, Borensztajn D, Jaegere A P D, Group N S. Ventilation practices in the neonatal intensive care unit: a cross-sectional study. *J. Pediatr*. 2010 Nov;157(5):767-71.e1-3.

[44] Tremblay L N, Slutsky A S. Ventilator-induced lung injury: from the bench to the bedside. *Intensive Care Medicine*. 2005 Oct 18;32(1):24–33.

[45] Tremblay L N, Slutsky A S. Ventilator-induced injury: from barotrauma to biotrauma. *Proc. Assoc. Am. Physicians*. 1998 Nov-Dec;110(6):482-8.

[46] te Pas A B, Wong C, Kamlin C O F, Dawson J A, Morley C J, Davis P G. Breathing Patterns in Preterm and Term Infants Immediately After Birth. *Pediatr. Res*. 2009 Mar;65(3):352–6.

[47] Kang L J, Cheung P Y, Pichler G, O'Reilly M, Aziz K, Schmölzer G M. Monitoring lung aeration during respiratory support in preterm infants at birth. *PLOS ONE*. 2014;9(7):e102729.

[48] Mian Q N, Cheung P Y, O'Reilly M, Pichler G, Os S van, Kushniruk K, Aziz K, Schmölzer G M. Spontaneously Breathing Preterm Infants Change in Tidal Volume to Improve Lung Aeration Immediately after Birth. *J. Pediatr*. 2015 May 18;167(2):274-278.e1.

[49] Mian Q N, Pichler G, Binder-Heschl C, O'Reilly M, Aziz K, Urlesberger B, Cheung P Y, Schmölzer G M. Tidal volumes in spontaneously breathing preterm infants supported with continuous positive airway pressure. *J. Pediatr*. 2014 Oct;165(4): 702-6.e1.

[50] Schmölzer G M, Kumar M, Pichler G, Aziz K, O'Reilly M, Cheung P Y. Non-invasive versus invasive respiratory support in preterm infants at birth: systematic review and meta-analysis. *BMJ*. 2013;347:f5980. doi: 10.1136/bmj.f5980.

[51] Keszler M. Novel Ventilation Strategies to Reduce Adverse Pulmonary Outcomes. *Clin. Perinatol*. 2022;49(1):219-242. doi: 10.1016/j.clp.2021.11.019.

[52] Lampland A L, Plumm B, Worwa C, Meyers P, Mammel M C. Bi-level CPAP does not improve gas exchange when compared with conventional CPAP for the treatment of neonates recovering from respiratory distress syndrome. *Arch. Dis. Child. Fetal Neonatal Ed*. 2015 Jan;100(1):F31-4.

[53] Victor S, Roberts S A, Mitchell S, Aziz H, Lavender T, Extubate Trial Group. Biphasic positive airway pressure or continuous positive airway pressure: a randomized trial. *Pediatrics*. 2016 Aug;138(2):e20154095

[54] Lemyre B, Davis P G, De Paoli A G, Kirpalani H. Nasal intermittent positive pressure ventilation (NIPPV) versus nasal continuous positive airway pressure (NCPAP) for preterm neonates after extubation. *Cochrane Database Syst. Rev.* 2017 Feb 1;2(2):CD003212.

[55] Wheeler K I, Klingenberg C, Morley C J, Davis P G. Volume-Targeted versus Pressure-Limited Ventilation for Preterm Infants: A Systematic Review and Meta-Analysis. *Neonatology.* 2011;100(3):219–27.

[56] Ali S K, Jayakar R V, Marshall A P, Gale T J, Dargaville P A. Preliminary study of automated oxygen titration at birth for preterm infants. *Arch. Dis. Child. Fetal Neonatal Ed.* 2022;fetalneonatal-2021-323486. doi: 10.1136/archdischild-2021-323486.

[57] Dargaville P A, Marshall A P, McLeod L, Salverda H H, Te Pas A B, Gale T J. Automation of oxygen titration in preterm infants: Current evidence and future challenges. *Early Hum. Dev.* 2021;162:105462. doi: 10.1016/j.earlhumdev.2021.105462.

Chapter 19

Biological Markers of Ventilator-Associated Lung Injury: Experimental and Clinical Studies

Ricardo Belo Quita*, MD
Pneumology Department,
Porto Hospital and University Center, Porto, Portugal

Abstract

Acute lung injury (ALI) and acute respiratory distress syndrome (ARDS) represent a continuum of injury that may arise from a number of primary insults. Localised injury may progress due to trauma from ventilation, a finding that has led to intense debate in the clinical and experimental literature over optimal ventilator management and directed increasing scientific interest toward the mechanisms of ventilator-induced lung injury (VILI).

The implementation of low tidal volume strategies has led to an improvement in outcomes, including reduction in mortality, however, mortality remains unacceptably high. One of the greatest difficulties in clinical studies has been distinguishing the underlying lung injury responsible for the patient's respiratory failure from the lung injury resulting from the particular settings of the mechanical ventilator.

Consequently, investigators have searched for biological markers that reflect specifically ventilator-attributable lung injury. Numerous biological markers associated with ventilator-associated lung injury were identified and new classes of potential biological markers and different

* Corresponding Author's Email: quitaricardo@gmail.com.

In: Ventilator Induced Lung Injury in Non-Invasive Ventilatory Support
Editor: Antonio M. Esquinas
ISBN: 979-8-88697-840-7

samples for their identification are being studied for their potential clinical role in ventilator lung injury.

Sufficient data exist to support the ongoing research of this markers on different kinds of biological samples. Currently some of these markers are already being targeted as a way to reduce inflammation and injury associated with VALI and VILI and to direct the most appropriate ventilatory modes, with positive and beneficial results. Further studies with larger sample size and preferentially with combination of clinical and experimental models are necessary to further strength this data.

Keywords: biological markers, ventilation, lung injury, inflammation

Introduction

Acute lung injury (ALI) and acute respiratory distress syndrome (ARDS) represent a continuum of injury that may arise from a number of primary insults [1]. Localised injury may progress due to trauma from ventilation, a finding that has led to intense debate in the clinical and experimental literature over optimal ventilator management and directed increasing scientific interest toward the mechanisms of ventilator-induced lung injury (VILI) [1]. The implementation of low tidal volume strategies has led to an improvement in outcomes, including reduction in mortality, however, mortality remains unacceptably high [2]. This chapter focus on lung injury due to invasive ventilation as most of the studies were performed on this setting.

One of the greatest difficulties in clinical studies has been distinguishing the underlying lung injury responsible for the patient's respiratory failure from the lung injury resulting from the settings of the mechanical ventilator. Consequently, investigators have searched for biological markers that reflect ventilator-attributable lung injury [2]. The term VILI refers to experimental models in which lung injury in induced directly by an injurious ventilation strategy. Ventilator-associated lung injury (VALI) refers to the additional injury imposed on a previously injured lung by mechanical ventilation in either the clinical setting or in experimental studies. [2] Researchers have used a variety of clinical and experimental models to determine the effects of mechanical ventilation or mechanical strain on the expression of biological markers of inflammation or injury [2].

Here we intend to summarize the most recent published literature relevant to this subject. Only potential markers of ventilator-attributable injury were considered.

Biologic Markers of Inflammation in Clinical Studies

The role of the innate immune response and inflammation in the pathogenesis of VILI has been widely studied in recent years [2]. Although some have suggested that inflammation may not be integral to the initiation of VILI, clearly a preponderance of data in this field support a major pathogenetic role for inflammation and lung neutrophil recruitment [2]. Most biological markers identified in plasma, serum, pulmonary edema fluid, and BAL fluid in experimental studies are cytokines and chemokines [2]. Although none of these mediators distinguishes ventilator-induced injury from other etiologies of lung injury, the temporal association between changes in levels of these proteins and changes in tidal volume or positive end-expiratory pressure (PEEP) along with inhibitor studies suggests a causative role [2].

The precise functional role of each mediator associated with ventilator-attributable lung injury is not completely understood [2]. In clinical studies, changes in levels of biological markers have been used primarily to identify ventilator-attributable injury rather than to study disease pathogenesis [2]. Elevated levels of circulating inflammatory markers such as soluble tumour necrosis factor-alpha receptors (sTNFRs) 1 and 2, and interleukins (IL-) 6 and 8, have all been associated with adverse outcomes in patients with ARDS, but lack specificity to VALI [3].

Ventilator-associated changes in levels of some biological markers have been correlated with patient outcomes, including duration of mechanical ventilation, organ failures, length of hospital stay, and mortality. As an example, soluble advanced glycation end-product (sRAGE) receptors are associated with alveolar type I cell injury, and elevated plasma levels correlated well with both severity of lung injury and increased mortality in patients ventilated at higher tidal volumes. The rate of decline in plasma levels of sRAGE was also greater in patients ventilated at a lower tidal volume. Similarly, elevated levels of plasma surfactant protein D, a product of alveolar type II cells, were associated with worse clinical outcomes in patients with lung injury, and the rise in levels of the marker was attenuated with low tidal volume ventilation [3].

Perhaps using both biological markers and clinical parameters together may offer a more sensitive and specific tool for detecting injury and predicting outcomes in patients with ARDS. A combination of IL-8, surfactant protein D and sTNFR-1, in addition to the Acute Physiology and Chronic Health Evaluation III (APACHE III) clinical risk score, improved the accuracy of risk prediction in ARDS when compared to clinical risk predictors alone [3].

Although some biological markers correlate well with injurious ventilation, none of the proposed biomarkers are specific for VALI. However, clinical risk prediction scores, genetic profiling, and biological markers of disease severity, when part of a wider lung protection strategy, could be useful to identify patients at risk of lung injury, to classify disease severity and outcomes, and to focus protective interventions [3].

Clinical Studies with Acute Lung Injury

Several clinical studies have reported changes in mediators or modulators of inflammation with mechanical ventilation [2]. Ranieri et al. [2, 4] studied 44 patients with ARDS, enrolled within 8h of initiation of mechanical ventilation. They were randomized to the conventional group (tidal volume 11+/-2ml/kg and PEEP 7+/-2) or a lower tidal volume (tidal volume 8+/-1 e PEEP 15+/-3); in both groups plateau pressure was of <35 cmH_2O. In 36h the blood and bronchial alveolar lavage values of Interleukin-1 receptor antagonist (IL- Ira), soluble tumour necrosis factor receptor-1 and 2 (sTNFR1 and 2) decreased in the lower tidal volume group. The bronchial alveolar lavage values of the conventional group increased, on the other hand. Additionally, the BAL value of IL1B, IL6, IL8, TNF alfa decreased in the group with less tidal volume but increased or remained unchanged in the other group. The same happened with the plasma values. A follow-up study [2, 5] of BAL neutrophils in samples collected from patients in this study demonstrated increased neutrophil activation in the samples from patients receiving mechanical ventilation with the conventional strategy.

The ARDS Network low tidal volume study [2, 6] which studied the effect of lower tidal volume, plateau pressure-limited ventilation compared with more conventional tidal volumes in 861 patients, has provided considerable data on several biological markers of VALI. In an analysis [2, 7] of samples from patients in this clinical trial showed that IL-6, IL-8, and IL-10 in blood were associated with increased risk of death independent of ventilation mode used. In the low tidal volume group, plasma levels of IL-6 decreased by 26% and IL-8 levels decreased by 12%, but levels of IL-10 did not change by the third study day. The odds ratio for mortality for plasma IL-6 level on day 3 of the study was 3.7 (95% confidence interval [CI], 2.7 to 5.7) per 10-fold increase in plasma IL-6 level. It is noteworthy that IL-6 and IL-8 levels did vary with clinical risk factor for ARDS and that factors such as infection could increase levels of these mediators. However, the authors calculated that the proportion of treatment effect in the low tidal volume group captured by day 3 IL-6 level was 30% (95% CI, 8 to 88%), suggesting that IL-6 may be a surrogate marker for mortality reduction attributable to low tidal volume ventilation [2].

Another analysis [2, 8] of 565 patients of the ARDS Network low tidal volume study, found that higher plasma surfactant protein (SP)-D levels at baseline were associated with an increased risk of death and that the low tidal volume strategy was further associated with a significant decrease in SP-D by study day 3. However, a previous report suggested that increased plasma SP-A levels are associated with fewer ventilator-free days and higher mortality in ARDS and ALI patients independent of tidal volume [2].

Parsons et al. [2, 9] showed that elevated plasma levels of sTNFR1 and sTNFR2 were associated with higher mortality in 377 patients with ARDS or ALI in the ARDS Network study. The odds ratios for mortality were 5.76 (95% CI, 2.63 to 12.6) for every 10-fold increase in plasma sTNFR1 and 2.58 (95% CI, 1.05 to 6.31) for every 10-fold increase in plasma sTNFR2. In agreement with the previous study by Ranieri et al., plasma sTNFR1 significantly decreased from enrolment to day 3 only in patients receiving mechanical ventilation with the low tidal volume strategy ($p = 0.037$) [2].

In companion *in vitro* studies, [2, 9] alveolar epithelial-like cells (A549 cells) released sTNFR1 but not sTNFR2 in response to stimulation with TNF-α, IL-1β, and interferon-γ. Therefore, sTNFR1 may be a marker of the alveolar epithelial response to inflammatory mediators in VALI [2].

Stuber et al. [2, 10] measured plasma IL-8, TNF-α, IL-1Ra, IL-10, and IL-6 in 12 patients with ALI before, during, and after changing tidal volume from 6 to 12 mL/kg for 1 h. Higher tidal volume ventilation induced a transient increase in plasma levels of each of these mediators and levels returned to baseline with tidal volume reduction. BAL levels of each of the cytokines increased throughout the study in the subset of patients who underwent BAL. Although the sampling of this study was small it may implicate higher tidal volumes as a contributor to increased plasma concentrations of these mediators [2].

Increased production of reactive oxygen species and NO derived reactive nitrogen species have also been implicated in the development and progression of ALI [2, 11], Gessner et al. [2, 12] found that exhaled breath condensate nitrite levels were strongly correlated with tidal volume in 28 ARDS patients ($r = 0.79$, $p = 0.001$). They further reported that the ratio of exhaled breath condensate nitrite to tidal volume correlated with lung injury severity as measured by Murray Lung Injury Severity Score ($r = 0.84$, $p = 0.0001$) [2, 13].

Therefore, the increase in nitrite for a given tidal volume was greater with more severe lung injury. These data support the hypothesis that more injured lungs are more susceptible to VALI and that nitrite levels increase with VALI [2].

Clinical Studies without Acute Lung Injury

Other clinical data have demonstrated that high tidal volume ventilation in the absence of pre-existing lung injury does not affect plasma cytokine and chemokine levels in patient [2]. Wrigge et al. [2, 14] reported that in 62 patients undergoing major thoracic or abdominal surgery randomized to ventilation with either 12 mL/kg or 6 mL/kg tidal volume and similar PEEP levels, ventilation strategy had no effect on plasma levels of TNF-α, IL-1β, IL-8, IL-6,or IL-10 after 3 h. In an earlier report, [2, 14] the same group found that among 39 patients who were American Society of Anaesthesiologists physical status I or II ventilation with either 15 mL/kg tidal volume without PEEP, 6 mL/kg without PEEP, or 6 mL/kg with PEEP had no effect on plasma levels of TNF-α, IL-1Ra, IL-6, or IL-12.

In contrast, Tsangaris et al. [2, 15] reported that among patients without lung injury who were placed on mechanical ventilation for airway protection, BAL levels of platelet-activating factor increased over 1 week of ventilation. Although platelet-activating factor has been shown to be a mediator of pulmonary edema no data regarding pulmonary edema or lung injury were reported in the study by Tsangaris et al. [2, 15].

Another biological marker in ongoing investigation is the soluble form of the receptor for advanced glycation end-products (sRAGE). In the attempt to evaluate the role of this marker Matthieu Jabaudon et al. [16] obtained plasma samples from 95 patients enrolled in a large randomized controlled trial of lung-protective ventilation for major abdominal surgery. Plasma levels of sRAGE were measured in duplicate with an enzyme-linked immunoassay on day 1, immediately after surgery, and on postoperative days 1, 3 and 7. Early postoperative plasma levels of sRAGE were significantly lower in the lung-protective ventilation group (n = 47) than in the non-protective ventilation group (n = 48) (mean (standard deviation), 1782 (836) vs 2171 (1678) pg/mL, respectively, P = 0.03). Intraoperative changes in plasma sRAGE were associated with postoperative hypoxemia and ARDS. This intraoperative decrease of sRAGE could reflect less epithelial injury and could potentially be used as a biological marker of VALI.

In a prospective, single-blind, randomized (1:1), parallel-group study by Mairi Ziaka et al., 18 critically ill patients with normal lungs were randomly assigned to receive mechanical ventilation with a tidal volume of either 6 mL/kg (low tidal volume) or 12 mL/kg (high tidal volume) during the first 4 days in the intensive care unit [17]. At baseline and at 24, 48, and 96 hours, exhaled breath condensate was collected to measure interleukin 1β, interleukin 10, tumor necrosis factor α, and total nitric oxide metabolites. Interleukin 1β levels in exhaled breath condensate were significantly increased at 24 hours compared with baseline in the high-tidal-volume group but not in the low-tidal-volume group. The interleukin 1β increase in the high-tidal-volume group was transient. Exhaled breath condensate levels of interleukin 1β, interleukin 10, tumor necrosis factor α, and total nitric oxide metabolites did not differ significantly between the high-tidal-volume and low-tidal-volume groups at any time point. Short-term mechanical ventilation with a tidal volume of 12 mL/kg may trigger inflammatory responses in the lungs of intensive care unit patients without preexisting lung injury [17]. More studies employing biological markers in exhaled breath condensate are needed to understand their clinical usefulness.

Canonical Wnt-signalling has been reported to serve an important role in the pathogenesis of VILI. Bioinformatics analysis revealed that canonical and non-canonical Wnt-signalling pathways were activated in VILI. A study [18] aimed to analyse the potential role of non-canonical Wnt-signalling in VILI pathogenesis demonstrated that 6 h of mechanical ventilation at low tidal volume (LTV; 6 ml/kg) or moderate tidal volume (MTV; 12 ml/kg) induced lung injury in sensitive A/J mice. Ventilation with MTV increased the protein levels of Wnt-induced secreted protein 1 (WISP1), Rho-associated protein kinase 1 (ROCK1), phosphorylated (p)-Ras homolog gene family, member A and p-C-Jun N-terminal kinase (JNK). Inhibition of ROCK1 by Y27632 and JNK by SP600125 attenuated MTV-induced lung injury and decreased the expression of proteins involved in non-canonical Wnt- signalling, including WISP1. In conclusion, non-canonical Wnt- signalling participates in VILI by modulating WISP1 expression, which has been previously noted as critical for VILI development [18].

In a prospective study, Magda Cepkova et al. [3] evaluated whether the institution of lung-protective positive pressure ventilation in spontaneously ventilating patients with ALI exacerbates pre-existing lung injury by using measurements of biomarkers of lung injury before and after intubation.

Twenty-five intubated, mechanically ventilated patients with ALI were enrolled. Serum samples were collected within 6 hours before intubation and at two different time points within the first 24 hours after intubation to measure the concentration of interleukin (IL)-6, IL-8, intercellular adhesion molecule 1 (ICAM-1), and von Willebrand factor (vWF).

The differences in biomarker levels before and after intubation were analysed using repeated measures analysis of variance and a paired t test with correction for multiple comparisons. Before endotracheal intubation, all of the biological markers (IL-8, IL-6, ICAM-1, and vWF) were elevated in the spontaneously breathing patients with ALI. After intubation and the institution of positive pressure ventilation (tidal volume 7 to 8 ml/kg per ideal body weight), none of the biological markers was significantly increased at either an early (3 ± 2 hours) or later (21 ± 5 hours) time point. However, the levels of IL-8 were significantly decreased at the later time point (21 ± 5 hours) after intubation.

During the 24-hour period after intubation, the PaO_2/FiO_2 (partial pressure of arterial oxygen/fraction of the inspired oxygen) ratio significantly increased, and the plateau airway pressure significantly decreased. This proved that the levels of IL-8, IL-6, vWF, and ICAM-1 are elevated in spontaneously ventilating patients with ALI prior to endotracheal intubation and that the institution of a lung-protective ventilation strategy with positive pressure ventilation does not further increase the levels of biological markers of lung injury.

Combined Experimental and Clinical Studies

Two reports have examined the roles of specific mediators in VALI in combined experimental and clinical studies. Imai et al. [2, 19] found that rabbits with acid-induced lung injury exposed to high tidal volume ventilation (12 mL/kg) had more severe pulmonary edema and increased epithelial apoptosis in the kidney and small intestine. Plasma from rabbits ventilated with high tidal volume induced apoptosis in renal tubule epithelial cells in culture and apoptosis in the cultured cells was significantly decreased by a Fas ligand blocking antibody.

In the clinical portion of the study, plasma levels of Fas ligand were found to correlate with higher plasma creatinine levels in 11 patients with ARDS. A previous study [2, 20] reported increased Fast ligand levels in pulmonary edema fluid from patients with ARDS. These data support the hypothesis that injurious ventilation leads to an increased circulating level of Fas ligand, which induces apoptosis in distal organs and potentially contributes to multiple organ failure [2].

Another study by Ye et al. [2, 21] induced lung injury in dogs with saline solution lavage and then ventilated the animals with a low tidal volume zero PEEP strategy for 6 h. Mice given intratracheal endotoxin were also ventilated with a high tidal volume of 17 mL/kg for 2 h. Lung tissue samples from the two animal models were analysed for gene expression using a gene chip microarray system. In both models, one gene demonstrating a significant increase in expression in the injured lungs was pre–B-cell colony enhancing factor (PBEF). BAL and serum levels of PBEF were found to be significantly higher in patients with ALI as compared to patients without lung injury. This series of experiments supports the hypothesis that both polymorphisms in the PBEF gene and PBEF levels are associated with an increased risk of ALI and VALI [2].

Experimental Studies of Ventilator-Attributable Lung Injury

Among the most studied biological markers in VILI and VALI are proinflammatory cytokines and chemokines.

Cytokines and Chemokines in Experimental Studies: Isolated Lung Models

Tremblay et al. [22] ventilated isolated nonperfused rat lungs for 2 h and found that high tidal volume, zero PEEP ventilation induced a much greater increase in airspace TNF-α, IL-1β, IL-6, IL-10, macrophage inflammatory protein (MIP)-2, and interferon-γ than lower tidal volume and high PEEP ventilation with similar peak inspiratory pressure or low tidal volume and zero PEEP ventilation. When rats were pre-treated with endotoxin 2 h before removal of the lungs and the ventilation procedure, levels of each of these mediators were significantly higher, with the exception of TNF-α in the high tidal volume group.

Ventilation of isolated mouse lungs with negative end-expiratory pressure has also been associated with increased BAL levels of TNF-α, affirming the hypothesis that excessively low lung volume ventilation and collapse of alveolar units may account for the observed changes in airspace cytokines. Veldhuizen et al. [23] found that in isolated mouse lungs, ventilation with a tidal volume of 20 mL/kg without PEEP resulted in significant increases in BAL levels of TNF-α and IL-6.

In Vivo Models of VALI

There are several reports of mechanical ventilation-attributable increases in cytokines and chemokines in whole-animal models [2].

Following acid aspiration induced lung injury in rats, higher tidal volumes are associated with greater increases in plasma and BAL TNF-α and MIP-2 [2, 24] and plasma IL-1β [2, 25] than acid injury alone or non-injurious ventilation. Others [26, 27, 28, 29] have reported comparable results in surfactant-depleted rats, rabbits, and pigs ventilated with high or low tidal volume or high-frequency oscillatory ventilation. Antibody blockade of TNF-α decreased histopathologic lung injury in surfactant-depleted rats [2, 28] while blockade of IL-1 with IL-1Ra attenuated lung injury after 8 h of ventilation in surfactant-depleted rabbits [2, 30]. In preterm lambs, higher lung volume ventilation with high PEEP resulted in greater increases in IL-1β, IL-6, and IL-8 but not TNF-α. [2, 5]. In preterm pigs, conventional tidal volume ventilation induced greater increases in leukotriene-B4 and IL-6 than high-frequency oscillatory ventilation or partial liquid ventilation; however, BAL levels of TNF-α were not different among the groups [2, 31].

Altemeier et al. [2, 32] pretreated rabbits with endotoxin before mechanical ventilation with a tidal volume of 15 mL/kg without PEEP for 8 h and found that endotoxin combined with mechanical ventilation resulted in significant increases in BAL levels of TNF-α, IL-8, growth-related oncogene-α, and MIP-1. Endotoxin or mechanical ventilation alone did not increase these cytokines. Others have also reported that endotoxin augments BAL and plasma levels of TNF-α following injurious ventilation [2, 33, 34].

In one study [2, 35] of VALI in rats, acid aspiration was followed by ventilation with either 12 mL/kg tidal volume and high or low PEEP, 6 mL/kg and high PEEP, or 3 mL/kg tidal volume and high PEEP. In the absence of acid injury, mechanical ventilation alone did not induce a measurable lung injury. Following acid injury, 4 h of mechanical ventilation with a tidal volume of 12 mL/kg resulted in more severe lung injury as measured by the severity of pulmonary edema and histopathologic and ultrastructural markers of cell injury. Higher tidal volume ventilation was also associated with higher airspace and plasma levels of RTI40, a rat type I pneumocyte-specific integral membrane protein. Furthermore, a reduction of tidal volume from 6 to 3 mL/kg resulted in a further significant reduction in plasma RTI40. Similarly, lung expression of SP-C messenger RNA, a type II cell specific protein, was lower following high-volume ventilation, although SP-C levels were not directly measured in the airspace fluid.

Paulo A. F. Magalhães et al. [36] compared the effects of assisted pressure support ventilation (PSV) with pressure-controlled ventilation (PCV) on lung function, histology and biological markers at two different PEEP levels in mild ARDS in rats. 35 Wistar rats received Escherichia coli lipopolysaccharide (LPS) intratracheally. After 24 h, the animals were sedated and randomly allocated to either PCV (n = 14) or PSV (n = 14) groups. Each group was further assigned to PEEP = 2 cmH_2O or PEEP = 5 cmH_2O. Tidal volume was kept constant (≈6 ml kg). Additional nonventilated animals (n = 7) were used as a control for postmortem analysis. In both PCV and PSV, peak transpulmonary pressure was lower, whereas E-cadherin tissue expression, which is related to epithelial integrity, was higher at PEEP = 5 cmH_2O than at PEEP = 2 cmH_2O. In PSV, PEEP = 5 cmH_2O compared with PEEP = 2 cmH_2O was associated with significantly reduced diffuse alveolar damage score [median (interquartile range), 11 (8.5 to 13.5) vs. 23 (19 to 26), $P = 0.005$] and expressions of IL-6 and CINC-1 ($P = 0.02$ for both), whereas surfactant protein-B mRNA expression increased ($P = 0.03$). These changes suggested less type II epithelial cell damage at a PEEP of 5 cmH_2O. Peak transpulmonary pressure correlated positively with IL-6 [Spearman's rho (ρ) = 0.62, $P = 0.0007$] and CINC-1 expressions ($\rho = 0.50$, $P = 0.01$) and negatively with E-cadherin expression ($\rho = -0.67$, $P = 0.0002$). During PSV, PEEP of 5 cmH_2O, but not a PEEP of 2 cmH_2O, reduced both lung damage and inflammatory markers while maintaining epithelial cell integrity.

Yu-Ling Dai et al. [37] studied a group of 15 pigs randomly allocated to 3 groups (n = 5 for each group): the control group, the VCV group and the ASV group. After left pneumonectomy, the VCV group was treated with the volume-control set to 20 ml/kg, and the ASV group with the mode set to achieve 60% of the minute ventilation of two lungs. results showed that VCV to the remaining lung caused increases in BALF IL-1b, IL-6, IL-8, and tumour necrosis factor-a, indicating significant airway inflammation, whereas ASV attenuated this inflammatory response. ASV also protected the lung from VILI, as indicated by a lower BALF protein concentration, a normal wet-to-dry weight ratio and a less severe lung injury score. There was a time dependent increases in EBC IL-1b and IL-6, which were consistent with the trend seen for serum cytokines. miRNAs are small non-coding RNAs that inhibit protein translation by directly promoting the cleavage of mRNA transcripts or by indirectly preventing mRNA access to the translational machinery. Several miRNAs, such as miR-17, miR-155, miR-429, miR34b-5p and miR-181a, have been shown to play critical roles in regulating inflammatory pathway in lung diseases [10]. This study results showed that VCV after pneumonectomy caused significant increases in the abundance of miR-144-5p, miR-449- 3p, miR-449b-5p and miR-451 and ASV resulted in significantly lower abundance of miR-144-5p, miR-449-3p and miR-451. It has been reported that the expression of miR-144-5p might be associated with inflammation responses [39]. This suggests that these miRNAs have potential roles as biomarkers of ventilator-associated lung injury.

J Y Wu et al. [38] investigated the potential role and possible mechanism of interleukin-10 (IL-10) and recombinant human keratinocyte growth factor-2 (rhKGF-2) in protecting anesthetized rats against VILI. A total of 50 male SD rats were randomly divided into 5 groups (N = 10 each): control, VILI, IL-10, rhKGF-2, and IL-10 + rhKGF-2. The VILI (model) group was generated via ventilation, with a tidal volume of 20 mL/kg. Rats in the IL-10 and rhKGF-2 groups received 8 mg/kg IL-10 and 5 mg/kg rhKGF-2, respectively, prior to ventilation. The rats in the IL-10 + rhKGF-2 group received both 8 mg/kg IL-10 and 5 mg/kg rhKGF-2 72 h before ventilation. The surfactant protein C (SP-C) mRNA expression in both IL-10 and rhKGF-2 groups was similar to that in the VILI group. However, this was significantly elevated in the combined treatment group ($P < 0.05$), indicating that IL-10 and rhKGF-2 could synergistically protect the lung tissue from VILI via the enhancement of SP-C mRNA expression in lung tissues. The protein assay showed a decreased level of infiltration and activation of inflammatory cells, in addition to increased expression of SP-C, thereby confirming the efficacy of this treatment in preventing VILI during anesthesia.

Shih-Hsing Yang et al. [39] tried to discover the role of IL-33 and its ST2 receptor in acute lung injury induced by mechanical ventilator. Male Wistar rats were intubated after tracheostomy and received ventilation at 10 cmH_2O of inspiratory pressure (PC10) by a G5 ventilator for 4 hours. The consequence of VILI by H&E stain showed inducing lung congestion and increasing the expression of pro-inflammatory cytokines such as TNF-α and IL-1β in the lung tissue homogenization, serum, and BALF, respectively. In addition, rats with VILI also exhibited high expression of IL-33 in lung tissues. Interestingly, the data showed that ST2L (membrane form) was highly accumulated in the membrane fraction of lung tissue in the PC10 group, but the ST2L in cytosol was dramatically decreased in the PC10 group. Conversely, the sST2 (soluble form) was slightly decreased both in the membrane and cytosol fractions in the PC10 group compared to the control group. In conclusion, these results demonstrated that ST2L translocation from the cytosol to the cell membranes of lung tissue and the down-expression of sST2 in both fractions can function as new biomarkers of VILI. Moreover, IL-33/ST2 signalling activated by mechanically responsive lung injury may potentially serve as a new therapy target [39].

Neutrophil gelatinase-associated lipocalin (NGAL) is a 25-kDa protein of the lipocalin superfamily and its presence was initially observed in activated neutrophils [40]. It has previously been demonstrated that the expression of NGAL is markedly increased in stimulated epithelia and is important in the innate immunological response to various pathophysiological conditions, including infection, cancer, inflammation and kidney injury. [40] Rui Xiao et al. [40] using a ventilator-associated lung injury model in mice demonstrated NGAL expression increased under all mechanical ventilation treatments. The increase was most prominent in the high peak inflation pressure and high-volume mechanical ventilation groups, where there was the greatest extent of lung injury. In addition, NGAL expression increased in a time-dependent manner under high-volume mechanical ventilation, consistent with the degree of lung injury. These findings suggested that NGAL may serve as a potential novel biomarker in ventilator-associated lung injury.

Pulmonary endothelial cell injury is central to the pathophysiology of acute lung injury [41], Mechanical ventilation can cause endothelial disruption and injury, even in the absence of pre-existing inflammation [41]. Platelet-endothelial cell adhesion molecule-1 is a transmembrane protein connecting adjacent endothelial cells. It was hypothesized that injurious mechanical ventilation will increase circulating lung endothelial-derived microparticles, defined as microparticles positive for platelet-endothelial cell adhesion molecule-1, which could serve as potential biomarkers and mediators of ventilator-induced lung injury.

To study this Nuria E Cabrera-Benítez et al. [41] performed a prospective randomized, controlled, animal investigation in which animals were randomly allocated to one of the three following ventilatory protocols for 4 hours: spontaneous breathing (control group), mechanical ventilation with low tidal volume (6 mL/kg), and mechanical ventilation with high tidal volume (20 mL/kg). In both mechanical ventilation groups, positive end-expiratory pressure of 2 cmH_2O was applied. When compared with low-tidal volume mechanical ventilation, high-tidal volume ventilation increased lung edema score and caused gas-exchange deterioration. These changes were associated with a marked increase of circulating endothelial-derived microparticles and a reduction of platelet-endothelial cell adhesion molecule-1 protein levels in the high-tidal volume lungs ($p < 0.0001$). Therefore, there is an endothelial-derived microparticle profile associated with disease-specific features of ventilator-induced lung injury and could serve both as a biomarker of acute lung injury [41].

Rongrong Ren et al. [42] studied phosphoprotein profiling of blood and tissue samples from ventilated and non-ventilated mice and key changes in protein levels and cell signalling during VILI. They detected activation of the PI3K/AKT, and mitogen activated protein kinase signalling pathways, in addition to changes in expression of cancer, inflammatory and cell-death related proteins as a response to mechanical ventilation. Focal adhesion-related protein levels and signalling pathways were also significantly altered in an injury model compared with control.

Another useful sample proved to be of value for biomarker research was urine. Weiwei Qin et al. [43] studied investigated potential urinary biomarkers to monitor the disease activity of ventilator-induced lung injury (VILI). Using, a label-free data-dependent acquisition (DDA) quantitative proteomics method to profile the urinary proteomes of VILI rats and the differential proteins were verified by parallel reaction monitoring (PRM)-targeted quantitative proteomics. Thirteen proteins were identified as candidate biomarkers for VILI by PRM validation. Among these PRM-validated proteins, AMPN, MEP1B, LYSC1, DPP4 and CYC were previously reported as lung-associated disease biomarkers. SLC31, MEP1A, S15A2, NHRF1, XPP2, GGT1, HEXA, and ATPB were newly discovered in this study. These results suggest that the urinary proteome might reflect the pathophysiological changes associated with VILI and that these differential proteins are potential urinary biomarkers for the activity of VILI.

To discover new biomarkers and mechanisms of VILI, Haoshu Ding et al. used isobaric Tag for Relative and Absolute Quantitation (iTRAQ)-based quantitative proteomics which were applied to identify differentially expressed proteins in mice treated with high tidal volume ventilation (HV), low tidal volume ventilation (LV) and lipopolysaccharide (LPS) [44]. A total of 14 dysregulated proteins showed the same change trend both in the LV and HV group and no change in the LPS group, and most importantly, the fold change of these proteins increased with the increase of volume ventilation, which indicates these proteins may be considered as potential markers specific for VILI. Ingenuity pathway analysis (IPA) canonical pathways analysis identified the top 4 canonical pathways, including the extrinsic prothrombin activation pathway, coagulation systems, the intrinsic prothrombin activation pathway, and the acute phase response, suggesting that these pathways, as associated with these proteins' expression, may be important therapeutic targets for reducing VILI. These findings will provide a new perspective for understanding the pathogenesis of VILI in the future [44].

A potential breath biomarker for ventilator-induced lung injury has also been subject to study. Lukas Martin Müller-Wirtz et al. [2] evaluated whether exhaled pentanal, a lipid peroxidation product, might be a useful breath biomarker for stretch-induced lung injury in rats. A total of 150 male Sprague-Dawley rats were investigated in 2 sub studies. The first randomly assigned 75 rats to 7 hours of mechanical ventilation at tidal volumes of 6, 8, 12, 16, and 20 mL·kg 1. The second included 75 rats. A reference group was ventilated at a tidal volume of 6 mL·kg-1 for 10 hours 4 interventional groups were ventilated at a tidal volume of 6 mL·kg-1 for 1 hour, and then for 0.5, 1, 2, or 3 hours at a tidal volume of 16 mL.kg-1 before returning to a tidal volume of 6 mL·kg-1 for additional 6 hours. Exhaled pentanal was monitored by multicapillary column-ion mobility spectrometry.

The first sub study included cytokine and leukocyte measurements in blood and bronchoalveolar fluid, histological assessment of the proportion of alveolar space, and measurements of myeloperoxidase activity in lung tissue. The second substudy included measurements of pentanal in arterial blood plasma, cytokine, and leukocyte concentrations in bronchoalveolar fluid, and cleaved caspase 3 in lung tissue.

Exhaled pentanal concentrations increased by only 0.5 ppb·h-1 (95% confidence interval [CI], 0.3-0.6) when rats were ventilated at 6 mL·kg-1. In contrast, exhaled pentanal concentrations increased substantially and roughly linearly at higher tidal volumes, up to 3.1 ppb·h-1 (95% CI, 2.3-3.8) at tidal volumes of 20 mL·kg-1. Exhaled pentanal increased at average rates between 1.0 ppb·h-1 (95% CI, 0.3-1.7) and 2.5 ppb·h-1 (95% CI, 1.4-3.6) after the onset of 16 mL·kg-1 tidal volumes and decreased rapidly by a median of 2 ppb (interquartile range [IQR], 0.9-3.2), corresponding to a 38% IQR, reduction when tidal volume returned to 6 mL·kg-1. Tidal volume, inspiratory pressure, and mechanical power were positively associated with pentanal exhalation. We can conclude that exhaled pentanal is a potential biomarker for early detection of ventilator-induced lung injury in rats.

Conclusion

During the past years, diverse biological markers associated with VALI or VILI had been previously identified in either clinical, experimental, or animal models. More recently, new classes of potential biological markers and different samples for their identification are being studied for their potential clinical role in ventilator lung injury. Sufficient data exists to support ongoing research of this markers on different kinds of biological samples. Currently some of this of these markers are already being targeted as a way to reduce inflammation and injury associated with VALI and VILI and to direct the most appropriate ventilatory modes, with positive and beneficial results.

Further studies with larger sample size and preferentially with combination of clinical and experimental models are necessary to further strength this data.

References

[1] Müller-Wirtz LM, Kiefer D, Maurer F, Floss MA, Doneit J, Hüppe T, Shopova T, Wolf B, Sessler DI, Volk T, Kreuer S, Fink T. Volutrauma Increases Exhaled Pentanal in Rats: A Potential Breath Biomarker for Ventilator-Induced Lung *Injury. Anesth Analg.* 2021 Jul 1;133(1):263-273. doi: 10.1213/ANE.0000000000005576. PMID: 33929393.

[2] James A, Frank, Polly E, Parsons and Michael A. Matthay. Pathogenetic Significance of Biological Markers of Ventilator Associated Lung Injury in Experimental and Clinical Studies. *Chest.* 2006 December; 130(6): 1906–1914. doi:10.1378/chest.130.6.1906.

[3] Magda Cepkova, Sandra Brady, Anil Sapru, Michael A Matthay & Gwynne Church. Biological markers of lung injury before and after the institution of positive pressure ventilation in patients with acute lung injury. *Crit Care* 10, R126 (2006). https://doi.org/10.1186/cc5037.

[4] Oeckler RA and Hubmayr RD. Ventilator-associated lung injury: a search for better therapeutic targets. *Eur Respir J* 2007; 30: 1216–1226. doi:10.1183/09031936.00104907.

[5] Salman D, Finney SJ, & Griffiths MJD. (2013). Strategies to reduce ventilator-associated lung injury (VALI). *Burns*, 39(2), 200–211. doi:10.1016/j.burns.2012.10.013.

[6] Ulrich Merz, Bernd Klosterhalfen, Martin Häusler, Melanie Kellinghaus, Thomas Peschgens, Helmut Hörnchen. Partial liquid ventilation reduces release of leukotriene B4 and interleukin-6 in bronchoalveolar lavage in surfactant-depleted newborn pigs. *Pediatr Res* 2002;51:183–189. [PubMed: 11809912].

[7] Ranieri VM, Suter PM, Tortorella C, De Tullio R, Dayer JM, Brienza A, Bruno F, Slutsky AS. Effect of mechanical ventilation on inflammatory mediators in patients with acute respiratory distress syndrome: a randomized controlled trial. *JAMA* 1999;282:54–61. [PubMed: 10404912].

[8] The Acute Respiratory Distress Syndrome Network. Ventilation with lower tidal volumes as compared with traditional tidal volumes for acute lung injury and the acute respiratory distress syndrome. *N Engl J Med* 2000;342:1301–1308. [PubMed: 10793162].

[9] Polly E Parsons, Mark D Eisner, B Taylor Thompson, Michael A Matthay, Marek Ancukiewicz, Gordon R Bernard, Arthur P Wheeler. Lower tidal volume ventilation and plasma cytokine markers of inflammation in patients with acute lung injury. *Crit Care Med* 2005;33:1–6. [PubMed:15644641].

[10] Eisner MD, Parsons P, Matthay MA, Ware L, Greene K. Plasma surfactant protein levels and clinical outcomes in patients with acute lung injury. *Thorax* 2003;58:983–988. [PubMed: 14586055].

[11] Polly E Parsons, Michael A Matthay, Lorraine B Ware, Mark D Eisner. Elevated plasma levels of soluble TNF receptors are associated with morbidity and mortality in patients with acute lung injury. *Am J Physiol Lung Cell Mol Physiol* 2004; 288:L426–L431. [PubMed: 15516488].

[12] Stüber F, Wrigge H, Schroeder S, Wetegrove S, Zinserling J, Hoeft A, Putensen C. Kinetic and reversibility of mechanical ventilation-associated pulmonary and systemic inflammatory response in patients with acute lung injury. *Intensive Care Med.* 2002 Jul;28(7):834-41. doi: 10.1007/s00134-002-1321-7. Epub 2002 Jun 15. PMID: 12122519.

[13] Gessner C, Hammerschmidt S, Kuhn H, Lange T, Engelmann L, Schauer J, Wirtz H. Exhaled breath condensate nitrite and its relation to tidal volume in acute lung injury. *Chest.* 2003 Sep;124(3):1046-52. doi: 10.1378/chest.124.3.1046. PMID: 12970036.

[14] Haddad I, Pitt, B, Matalon S. Nitric oxide and lung injury. In: Fishman, AP., editor. *Pulmonary Diseases and Disorders.* New York, NY: McGraw-Hill; 1996. p. 337-346.

[15] Wrigge H, Uhlig U, Zinserling J, Behrends-Callsen E, Ottersbach G, Fischer M, Uhlig S, Putensen C. The effects of different ventilatory settings on pulmonary and systemic inflammatory responses during major surgery. *Anesth Analg.* 2004 Mar;98(3):775-81, table of contents. doi: 10.1213/01.ane.0000100663.11852.bf. PMID: 14980936.

[16] Tsangaris I, Lekka ME, Kitsiouli E, Constantopoulos S, Nakos G. Bronchoalveolar lavage alterations during prolonged ventilation of patients without acute lung injury. *Eur Respir J.* 2003 Mar;21(3):495-501. doi: 10.1183/09031936.03.00037902. PMID: 12662008.

[17] Jabaudon M, Futier E, Roszyk L, Sapin V, Pereira B, Constantin JM. Association between intraoperative ventilator settings and plasma levels of soluble receptor for advanced glycation end-products in patients without pre-existing lung injury. *Respirology.* 2015 Oct;20(7):1131-8. doi: 10.1111/resp.12583. Epub 2015 Jun 29. PMID: 26122046.

[18] Ziaka M, Makris D, Fotakopoulos G, Tsilioni I, Befani C, Liakos P, Zygoulis P, Zakynthinos E. High-Tidal-Volume Mechanical Ventilation and Lung Inflammation in Intensive Care Patients with Normal Lungs. *Am J Crit Care*. 2020 Jan 1;29(1):15-21. doi: 10.4037/ajcc2020161. PMID: 31968080.

[19] Xia YF, Chang J, Yang JF, Ouyang W, Pitt B, Billiar T, Zhang LM. Non-canonical Wnt signaling contributes to ventilator-induced lung injury through upregulation of WISP1 expression. *Int J Mol Med*. 2019 Mar;43(3):1217-1228. doi: 10.3892/ijmm.2019.4067. Epub 2019 Jan 17. PMID: 30664165; PMCID: PMC 6365043.

[20] Albertine KH, Soulier MF, Wang Z, Ishizaka A, Hashimoto S, Zimmerman GA, Matthay MA, Ware LB. Fas and fas ligand are up-regulated in pulmonary edema fluid and lung tissue of patients with acute lung injury and the acute respiratory distress syndrome. *Am J Pathol*. 2002 Nov;161(5):1783-96. doi: 10.1016/S0002-9440(10)64455-0. PMID: 12414525; PMCID: PMC1850801.

[21] Ye SQ, Simon BA, Maloney JP, Zambelli-Weiner A, Gao L, Grant A, Easley RB, McVerry BJ, Tuder RM, Standiford T, Brower RG, Barnes KC, Garcia JG. Pre-B-cell colony-enhancing factor as a potential novel biomarker in acute lung injury. *Am J Respir Crit Care Med*. 2005 Feb 15;171(4):361-70. doi: 10.1164/rccm.200404-563OC. Epub 2004 Dec 3. PMID: 15579727.

[22] Tremblay L, Valenza F, Ribeiro SP, Li J, Slutsky AS. Injurious ventilatory strategies increase cytokines and c-fos m-RNA expression in an isolated rat lung model. *J Clin Invest*. 1997 Mar 1;99(5):944-52. doi: 10.1172/JCI119259. PMID: 9062352; PMCID: PMC507902.

[23] Veldhuizen RA, Slutsky AS, Joseph M, McCaig L. Effects of mechanical ventilation of isolated mouse lungs on surfactant and inflammatory cytokines. Eur *Respir J*. 2001 Mar;17(3):488-94. doi: 10.1183/09031936.01.17304880. PMID: 11405530.

[24] Chiumello D, Pristine G, Slutsky AS. Mechanical ventilation affects local and systemic cytokines in an animal model of acute respiratory distress syndrome. *Am J Respir Crit Care Med* 1999;160:109– 116. [PubMed: 10390387].

[25] Frank JA, Matthay MA. Science review: mechanisms of ventilator-induced injury. Crit Care 2003;7:233–241. [PubMed: 12793874].

[26] Imai Y, Nakagawa S, Ito Y, Kawano T, Slutsky AS, Miyasaka K. Comparison of lung protection strategies using conventional and high-frequency oscillatory ventilation. *J Appl Physiol* (1985). 2001 Oct;91(4):1836-44. doi: 10.1152/jappl. 2001.91.4.1836. PMID: 11568170.

[27] Steinberg JM, Schiller HJ, Halter JM, Gatto LA, Lee HM, Pavone LA, Nieman GF. Alveolar instability causes early ventilator-induced lung injury independent of neutrophils. *Am J Respir Crit Care Med*. 2004 Jan 1;169(1):57-63. doi: 10.1164/ rccm.200304-544OC. PMID: 14695106.

[28] Imai Y, Kawano T, Iwamoto S, Nakagawa S, Takata M, Miyasaka K. Intratracheal anti-tumor necrosis factor-alpha antibody attenuates ventilator-induced lung injury in rabbits. *J Appl Physiol* (1985). 1999 Aug;87(2):510-5. doi: 10.1152/jappl.1999. 87.2.510. PMID: 10444606.

[29] Takata M, Abe J, Tanaka H, Kitano Y, Doi S, Kohsaka T, Miyasaka K. Intraalveolar expression of tumor necrosis factor-alpha gene during conventional and high-

frequency ventilation. *Am J Respir Crit Care Med.* 1997 Jul;156(1):272-9. doi: 10.1164/ajrccm.156.1.9607072. PMID: 9230760.

[30] Narimanbekov IO, Rozycki HJ. Effect of IL-1 blockade on inflammatory manifestations of acute ventilator-induced lung injury in a rabbit model. *Exp Lung Res* 1995;21:239–254. [PubMed: 7774527].

[31] Naik AS, Kallapur SG, Bachurski CJ, Jobe AH, Michna J, Kramer BW, Ikegami M. Effects of ventilation with different positive end-expiratory pressures on cytokine expression in the preterm lamb lung. *Am J Respir Crit Care Med.* 2001 Aug 1;164(3):494-8. doi: 10.1164/ajrccm.164.3.2010127. PMID: 11500356.

[32] Altemeier WA, Matute-Bello G, Frevert CW, Kawata Y, Kajikawa O, Martin TR, Glenny RW. Mechanical ventilation with moderate tidal volumes synergistically increases lung cytokine response to systemic endotoxin. *Am J Physiol Lung Cell Mol Physiol.* 2004 Sep;287(3):L533-42. doi: 10.1152/ajplung.00004.2004. Epub 2004 May 14. Erratum in: *Am J Physiol Lung Cell Mol Physiol.* 2005 Apr;288(4): L771. PMID: 15145786.

[33] Haitsma JJ, Uhlig S, Göggel R, Verbrugge SJ, Lachmann U, Lachmann B. Ventilator-induced lung injury leads to loss of alveolar and systemic compartmentalization of tumor necrosis factor-alpha. Intensive *Care Med.* 2000 Oct;26(10):1515-22. doi: 10.1007/s001340000648. PMID: 11126266.

[34] Murphy DB, Cregg N, Tremblay L, Engelberts D, Laffey JG, Slutsky AS, Romaschin A, Kavanagh BP. Adverse ventilatory strategy causes pulmonary-to-systemic translocation of endotoxin. Am J Respir Crit Care Med. 2000 Jul;162(1):27-33. doi: 10.1164/ajrccm.162.1.9908110. Erratum in: *Am J Respir Crit Care Med* 2002 Dec 1;166(11):1517. PMID: 10903215.

[35] Frank JA, Gutierrez JA, Jones KD, Allen L, Dobbs L, Matthay MA. Low tidal volume reduces epithelial and endothelial injury in acid-injured rat lungs. *Am J Respir Crit Care Med.* 2002 Jan 15;165(2):242-9. doi: 10.1164/ajrccm.165.2.2108087. PMID: 11790662.

[36] Magalhães PAF, Padilha GA, Moraes L, Santos CL, Maia LA, Braga CL, Duarte MDCMB, Andrade LB, Schanaider A, Capellozzi VL, Huhle R, Gama de Abreu M, Pelosi P, Rocco PRM, Silva PL. Effects of pressure support ventilation on ventilator-induced lung injury in mild acute respiratory distress syndrome depend on level of positive end-expiratory pressure: A randomised animal study. *Eur J Anaesthesiology.* 2018 Apr;35(4):298-306. doi: 10.1097/EJA.0000000000000763. PMID: 29324568.

[37] Tokioka H, Saito S, Kosaka F. Comparison of pressure support ventilation and assist control ventilation in patients with acute respiratory failure. *Intensive Care Med.* 1989;15(6):364-7. doi: 10.1007/BF00261494. PMID: 2681311.

[38] Dai YL, Hsu RJ, Huang HK, Huang TW, Tsai WC, Chang H, Lan CC, Huang KL. Adaptive support ventilation attenuates postpneumonectomy acute lung injury in a porcine model. *Interact Cardiovasc Thorac Surg.* 2020 Nov 1;31(5):718-726. doi: 10.1093/icvts/ivaa157. PMID: 33051664.

[39] Wu JY, Xiong ZH, Xiong GZ, Ding FQ, Lei J, Lu S, Li Y, He GM, Zhao LL, Liu ZJ. Protective effect of interleukin-10 and recombinant human keratinocyte growth

factor-2 on ventilation-induced lung injury in rats. *Genet Mol Res.* 2015 Dec 2;14(4):15642-51. doi: 10.4238/2015. December.1.16. PMID: 26634532.

[40] Yang SH, Lin JC, Wu SY, Huang KL, Jung F, Ma MC, Wang Hsu GS, Jow GM. Membrane translocation of IL-33 receptor in ventilator induced lung injury. *PLoS One.* 2015 Mar 27;10(3): e0121391. doi: 10.1371/journal.pone.0121391. PMID: 25815839; PMCID: PMC4376768.

[41] Xiao R, Chen R. Neutrophil gelatinase-associated lipocalin as a potential novel biomarker for ventilator-associated lung injury. *Mol Med Rep.* 2017 Jun;15(6):3535-3540. doi: 10.3892/mmr.2017.6442. Epub 2017 Apr 7. PMID: 28393227; PMCID: PMC5436233.

[42] Cabrera-Benítez NE, Valladares F, García-Hernández S, Ramos-Nuez Á, Martín-Barrasa JL, Martínez-Saavedra MT, Rodríguez-Gallego C, Muros M, Flores C, Liu M, Slutsky AS, Villar J. Altered Profile of Circulating Endothelial-Derived Microparticles in Ventilator-Induced Lung Injury. Crit Care Med. 2015 Dec;43(12): e551-9. doi: 10.1097/CCM.0000000000001280. Erratum in: *Crit Care Med.* 2016 Mar;44(3): e180. PMID: 26308427.

[43] Ren R, Ruan Z, Ding H, Du J, Yu W. Phosphoproteome profiling provides insight into the mechanisms of ventilator-induced lung injury. *Exp Ther Med.* 2020 Jun;19(6):3627-3633. doi: 10.3892/etm.2020.8634. Epub 2020 Apr 1. PMID: 32346427; PMCID: PMC7185165.

[44] Qin W, Zhang X, Chen L, Li Q, Zhang B, Sun L, Han W. Differential urine proteome analysis of a ventilator-induced lung injury rat model by label-free quantitative and parallel reaction monitoring proteomics. *Sci Rep.* 2021 Nov 2;11(1):21446. doi: 10.1038/s41598-021-01007-w. PMID: 34728735; PMCID: PMC8563714.

[45] Ding H, Wang Y, Dong W, Ren R, Mao Y, Deng X. Proteomic Lung Analysis of Mice with Ventilator-Induced Lung Injury (VILI) Using iTRAQ-Based Quantitative Proteomics. *Chem Pharm Bull* (Tokyo). 2018;66(7):691-700. doi: 10.1248/cpb.c17-00844. PMID: 29962452.

Chapter 20

Monitoring Techniques: The Pressure/Volume Curve

Riccardo La Rosa, MD
Savino Spadaro, MD, PhD
and Gaetano Scaramuzzo*, MD
Department of Translational Medicine, University of Ferrara, Ferrara, Italy

Abstract

Mechanical ventilation (MV) is a key support in patients with respiratory failure, but it can expose injured lungs to further damage. Pressure monitoring during tidal breathing is part of the clinical monitoring of MV. The pressure-volume (P/V) curve is a simple, reliable, and bedside monitoring technique that explores changes in the respiratory system compliance along a wide range of pressures. The P/V usually has a sigmoidal shape, with two main changes in compliance, described as inflection points. This peculiar behavior of the respiratory system during tidal breathing has been suggested to reflect alveolar recruitment and, eventually, overdistention.

In ARDS patients, where risk of ventilator-induced lung injury (VILI) is particularly high, the P/V shape can be used to explore safety thresholds for airway pressures. On one hand, the lower inflection point (LIP) could help to titrate the end-expiratory pressure (PEEP), avoiding cyclic de-recruitment and therefore atelectrauma, while the upper inflection point (UIP) could indicate the threshold for plateau pressure to avoid alveolar overdistention.

---

* Corresponding Author's Email: gaetano.scaramuzzo@unife.it.

In: Ventilator Induced Lung Injury in Non-Invasive Ventilatory Support
Editor: Antonio M. Esquinas
ISBN: 979-8-88697-840-7

Ventilation along the range of pressures at which the respiratory system shows linear compliance can represent a strategy to reduce VILI in ARDS patients. Nevertheless, the P/V curve may represent the average behavior of the lung, and it is possible that may not reflect the entire parenchyma, since a regional behavior should not be underestimated. Although P/V curve has proven to be a practical bedside tool, its role in MV titration is still uncertain.

Keywords: pressure/volume, lung mechanics, VILI, mechanical ventilation

Introduction

The pressure-volume (P/V) curve has been used as a bedside maneuver to evaluate the mechanical behavior of the lung during passive inflation and deflation. Invasive mechanical ventilation (MV), indeed, changes how pressure and volumes are distributed into the lung. When passively inflated, the lung pressure changes and progressively increases proportionally to the inflated volume. The relationship between the volume inflated and the pressure can be described graphically as a curve, that takes therefore the name of pressure/volume curve (P/V curve). This can be done both for inspiration and expiration (inspiratory and expiratory limb), since the two curves do not necessary overlap each other, for the different behavior of the lung during inspiration and expiration.

The relationship between pressure and volume is complex and can be altered by gas flow and acceleration, the presence of the resistive components (airways and ventilatory circuit) or of any muscular activity, which is the reason why the maneuver is performed in sedated and paralyzed patients. Many methods have been described to obtain a P/V curve. Whatever method is chosen, if the inflation is achieved slowly the influence of gas flow acceleration and of the resistive components become mathematically negligible [1]. We usually refer to this specific P/V curve as the "quasi-static" curves since it is performed in dynamic conditions but reducing the influence of the dynamic components. Furthermore, the curve is usually built by recording pressure and volumes at airway opening.

In this case, we are simultaneously assessing the change of both lungs and chest wall, and the latter may play a variable and unpredictable role in the respiratory system compliance. To be precise, this P/V curve should be called therefore respiratory system P/V curve. Since the calculation of the lung pressure-volume curve would require the use of pleural pressure or of one surrogate (i.e., esophageal pressure), the respiratory system P/V curve is the one usually performed in clinical practice. In this case, we assume that the respiratory system behavior represents a good surrogate of the lung's one, allowing the description of lung performance at different pressures and in different conditions with less invasiveness [2].

The P/V curve has been used to describe both healthy and injured lungs and the shape of the curve and the curvature points may assume a specific connotation in pathological conditions such as ARDS, COPD, and pulmonary fibrosis [1, 3].

Building a P/V Curve

In clinical practice, the most widely used methods to build a P/V curve are: the super-syringe method, the constant-flow method, and the multiple-occlusion method. All three have in common a slow and progressive inflation of volume into a passive system (i.e., the respiratory system), being the patient fully paralyzed and mechanically ventilated via endotracheal tube (ETT).

The super-syringe method begins with a connection between a large volume syringe and the ETT, once the respiratory system is allowed to reach its relaxed volume. A stepwise inflation is then performed, generally increasing volume by 100 mL at each step and allowing a 2-3 second pause to reach equilibrium in pressures. Pressure measured at each volume is plotted, so that an inflation curve can be drawn. For safety reasons, maneuver usually stops when airway pressure reaches 30–40 cmH_2O. Thereafter, a progressive deflation, analogous to the previous steps, is performed to delineate the expiratory limb of the P/V curve. The main advantage of this method indeed lies in the possibility to realize both inspiratory and expiratory curves. On the other hand, the disconnection of the patient from the ventilator, the desaturation risk, the change in temperature and humidity and the compression of gases during the procedure constitute potential disadvantages to this maneuver, which is therefore seldom used in clinical setting nowadays.

The multiple occlusion method allows the construction of a quasi-static P/V curve by performing inspiratory pauses at incremental tidal volumes, so that single points of the curve can be plotted. In this case, ventilator disconnection is not necessary, and both sides of the loop can be drawn (inflation and deflation phase), starting from end expiratory volume. However, it is possible that progressive inspiratory pauses determine lung recruitment that can alter the pressure-volume relation [4]. Moreover, absolute volume is not measured as measurements are performed intermittently and over many breaths.

The constant-flow method is commonly used in clinical practice, also because some modern ventilators can generate it automatically. As the name suggests, a constant flow is applied to the respiratory system, so that inflation begins from end-expiratory volume and rises slowly without intermediate pauses. To ensure that gas flow itself does not interfere in total pressure by rising airway resistance, a slow flow, usually around or below 5 L/min, is chosen [1]. This allows the construction of a reliable inspiratory P/V curve, whereas expiratory curve is usually not achieved with this maneuver. More recently, some ventilators offer the opportunity to slow down expiration to also assess the expiratory limb of the P/V curve, generating an automatic expiratory P/V loop.

The P/V curve maneuver can expose the patients to possible procedure-related risks, such as hypoxemia and hemodynamic changes (mainly in hypovolemic patients for a decreased venous return) and therefore a certain expertise in preventing and anticipating these possible events is required.

Interpretation P/V Curve

Inspiratory Limb

Independently from the method used, the pressure-volume curve represents a non-linear relation between increasing/decreasing pressure (represented on X-axis) and increasing/decreasing volume (Y-axis). The best fit to describe what happens to lung volumes when pressure is applied to respiratory system seems to be a sigmoidal curve [5]. Therefore, the inspiratory limb of the curve may be simplified into three segments and two inflection points, the lower and the upper inflection point (LIP and UIP, respectively).

In the first and last section of the P/V curve, the pressure increase corresponds to a low increase in volume. Given that compliance is defined as $\Delta V/\Delta P$, these regions of the P/V curve correlate to low-compliance state of the system, namely present at the two extremities of the curve. When inflation starts at low lung volumes, respiratory system shows a lower tendency to be expanded in response to the pressure applied. This initial inertia may be related to the reduced amount of parenchyma (derecruited lung) participating to volume expansion. Above a certain pressure, the slope of the curve changes and the intermediate segment starts; this section shows almost linear development. Being the slope once again determined by the compliance of the system, this region of the P/V curve shows therefore the best compliance [6]. This segment changes its slope at the UIP.

The upper extreme of inspiratory P/V curve shows again a lower compliance, as stated before, and that can relate to the behavior of lungs when over-inflation occurs. That is, a further increase in volume is possible, but at cost of much higher airway pressure. This is particularly relevant in ARDS, where both tendency to decruitment and to hyperinflation are highly present, due to the edema and to the parenchyma available for ventilation ("*baby lung*") [5, 7]. The inflection points can be found at different pressure levels among patients and during the disease, and this make the P/V curve a good monitoring technique to assess the patient's respiratory system properties and evaluate it over time and between different ventilatory modes (e.g., different PEEP levels). Despite this, the interpretation of the inflection points has proven challenging.

From a mathematical point of view, an inflection point of the curve would be from which the sigmoid changes its concavity. Clinical interest in time has focused on two points of the curve, defined as lower inflection point (LIP) and upper inflection point (UIP).

Gattinoni et al. [3] studying ARDS patients, described a "P_{flex}" referring to the point, in the lower part of the P/V, where two different linear compliances meet. In other words, two compliance lines are drawn, for the low compliance phase at the beginning of inflation and for the higher compliance phase at higher volume, respectively. These two linear compliances meet at a pressure point, which has been related to the pressure at which lung parenchyma has been sufficiently recruited and better complies to further imposed volume. This is what we now commonly refer to as lower inflection point, or LIP. Parenchymal recruitment, though, may be better described over a wider range of pressures, rather than on a single point of the curve, as a mathematical model of the P/V curve suggests [8].

Similarly, the upper branch of the curve offers a change in linear compliance that can be plotted as a point of pressure, known as upper inflection point (UIP), which has been felt as a mark of overdistention, since alveolar recruitment has already reached its plateau. Again, this was clinically highlighted in ARDS patients, where ventilation was found to happen at higher points of the P/V curve, causing alveolar strain, and suggesting that safer ventilation for these patients should target lower volumes, as ARDS network trials widely demonstrated [7, 9].

Expiratory Limb

The expiratory limb of the P/V curve, in time, has been less studied than the inspiratory one and uncertainties on its interpretation exist. Albaiceta et al. [7] studied P/V deflation, comparing its shape and characteristics between patients with pulmonary and extrapulmonary ARDS. They also performed maneuvers while measuring esophageal pressure, allowing comparison of chest wall, transpulmonary and global pressure-volume curves. The rationale behind measurement of expiratory P/V curve lies in the fact that PEEP is an expiratory phenomenon, avoiding alveolar collapse, so that deflation limb of the P/V curve may represent a better tool for PEEP setting. Indeed, by measuring transpulmonary pressure during deflation P/V maneuver, it was possible to observe different lung mechanics whether ARDS was of pulmonary (ARDSp) or extrapulmonary (ARDSe) origin. ARDSp shows a smaller lung capacity, and a larger derecruited volume during the expiratory phase, prompting to a higher PEEP requirement.

Clinical Relevance of P/V Monitoring

Monitoring the pressure/volume relation in mechanically ventilated patients can be useful to better understanding of how respiratory system changes its behavior during pulmonary disease. Acute respiratory distress syndrome (ARDS) constitutes a pivotal example of how ventilatory strategies can make a difference in patient outcome. Inflammatory insults to lung parenchyma, which represent a pathophysiologic hallmark in ARDS, expose alveoli to an increased mechanical stress. Mechanical ventilation improves gas exchanges and relieve muscular effort but exposes to ventilator-induced lung injury (VILI), especially when higher pressure and volumes are necessary to maintain adequate gas tension in blood. Thus, P/V has been proposed as a monitoring tool to reveal pressure-volume relation in ARDS lungs.

In ARDS the P/V curve shows a downward shift, indicating total lung capacity reduction, and, more importantly, global compliance seems reduced, which is coherent to modifications that take place during inflammatory remodeling of the lung [10]. The different shapes of the P/V curve in ARDS suggests that, when setting mechanical ventilation, it is challenging to choose and maintain a range of airway pressures to keep sufficient alveolar recruiting, while avoiding overdistention and therefore lung trauma.

Amato et al. [9] used the lower inflection point of the P/V as a reference for correct end-expiratory pressure (PEEP) titration in ARDS patients. Assuming that below LIP alveolar recruitment is insufficient to ensure adequate gas exchanges, PEEP in this study was set to be 2 cmH_2O higher than estimated LIP. Therefore, during expiratory phase, airway pressure does not fall below the lower inflection point, preventing alveolar cyclic de-recruitment.

The upper inflection point has been interpreted as a pressure level at which lung starts to be overstretch, potentially acting therefore as an indicator of barotrauma. When ventilation occurs at pressures higher than the UIP (e.g., higher tidal volumes and/or higher PEEP), stress and strain alter lung structure, overcoming a structural threshold for overdistention and damage, as animal model have shown [11]. An upper inflection point is identifiable in most ARDS patients and occurs at a much lower volume than in normal lungs [12], confirming altered compliance and stress tolerance. Therefore, a "safety range" of airway pressure during MV has been logically set between LIP and UIP, so that alveolar damage is minimized, without compromising oxygen delivery during ventilation.

Caveats and Future Perspectives

P/V curves of the respiratory system represent an interesting and readily accessible tool to assess lung response to pressure and volume stress. Although its physiological relevance seems clear, the role of the P/V in clinical decisions remains controversial. In fact, discussion is still open on how P/V should be interpreted in clinical context, and how it should affect clinical management of mechanically ventilated patients.

An interesting point of view on P/V behavior comes from a mathematical study by Hickling et al. [8]. In this model, alveolar units are characterized by different "threshold opening pressures" (TOP), meaning different trans-alveolar pressures that have to be exceeded in order to recruit parenchyma. Alveolar units show low compliance until trans-alveolar pressure reaches and surpasses their TOP, then their compliance varies linearly as their volume increases.

The sigmoidal shape of P/V, as previously described, is best depicted in this mathematical model when TOP is not a single value but is distributed in a wide range of pressures. The lower values of TOP seem to modify the position of LIP, whereas the higher values of threshold opening pressure affect the UIP of the curve. It is hence possible to argue that pressure-volume curve, as we classically draw it, represents the global behavior of lung parenchyma during inflation – that is what Hickling proposed as "mean P/V slope". Therefore, inflection points obtained from classical P/V may not be representative of all alveolar regions. Both mathematical models from Venegas and Hickling suggest that alveolar recruitment happens on a broad distribution along the curve [5, 8] depending on regional behavior of alveoli.

Recent evidence shows that regional pressure-volume curves can be described [13]. In this case, electrical impedance tomography (EIT) was performed during evaluation of global P/V curves (PVg) in 41 patients with AHRF or ARDS (all supine, deeply sedated and paralyzed during MV). EIT permits to explore regional behavior of lung during inflation, by showing how impedance (higher impedance means higher presence of air) changes in small chunks of volume in a tomographic section of lungs.

By plotting regional impedance variation (ΔZ) against pressure variation (during slow-flow P/V curve), it was possible to obtain 729 regional PVs (PVr) and describe the behavior of dependent and non-dependent lung during inflation. This analysis showed that regional behavior differs from what global P/V curve usually shows.

Namely, a gradient of regional lower inflection points was found from the non-dependent to the dependent lung. Moving toward the dependent lung (i.e., dorsal region when patient is supine) the LIP increases significantly and PVg tends to underestimate this value. Since the dependent lung is most exposed during mechanical ventilation to intra-cycle opening and closure, adjusting PEEP on global LIP may not be sufficient to ensure the pressure needed to start inflating these regions. The maximum LIP in regional curves should hence represent the minimum pressure that prevents closure of the most dorsal lung.

Moreover, relevant differences exist between global UIP and regional values of upper inflection point. Non-dependent lung shows lower values of UIP, suggesting that this region may be exposed to overstretch and damage at lower threshold than expected with PVg. In other words, global P/V may not provide a reliable "overdistention threshold", being the non-dependent lung already overstretching at pressures below global UIP (Figure 1).

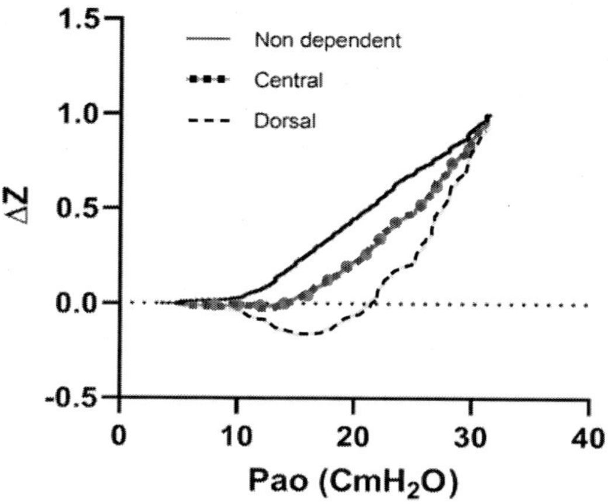

ΔZ = variation of impedance; Pao = airway opening pressure. The 3 curves represent the behavior of 3 different lung regions, i.e., the non-dependent (black), central (dark grey) and dependent lung (light grey). It can be noted how the lower inflection point moves to higher values of pressure going from the non-dependent to the dependent lung region.

Figure 1. Example of EIT derived regional pressure volume curves in an ARDS patient.

These results suggest that traditional P/V curve could provide partial information on how lung behaves during inflation, therefore giving an incomplete tool to titrate mechanical ventilation settings.

Even more so, controversial data emerged recently from Chen et al. [14], in studies where P/V curve was recorded in ARDS patients. They recorded a slow-flow PVC curve at different levels of PEEP. A significant quota of their population showed an extremely slow slope at the beginning of the inflation curve, almost corresponding to the ventilatory circuit compliance measured at the same PEEP level. At a certain pressure, the P/V curve abruptly changes its compliance, as if small airways remain closed, with no communication with alveoli, until sufficient pressure for airway opening (i.e., airway opening pressure, AOP) is reached. When integrating findings from this study group, it is tempting to say that in ARDS there is an unexpectedly high prevalence of airway closure, and opening pressure is not strictly related to a positive trans-alveolar pressure, but rather to a threshold pressure necessary to re-establish communication between alveoli and main airway.

Overall, recent evidence is therefore expanding and challenging our knowledge on the P/V curve. P/V curves represent a readily available, bedside tool to titrate pressure and tidal volume during ventilation, providing information on the global behavior of lung per each inflation cycle. On the other hand, avoiding parenchymal damage during MV has proven a challenge: changes and inhomogeneities in lung tissue [15] during ARDS makes it difficult to uniformly recruit alveolar units while avoiding overdistention or cyclic collapse of some units.

The linear part described in classical P/V curve seems to be a compromise between ventilation of dependent and non-dependent lung [14], but compromise may not be the best option for all patients during invasive mechanical ventilation [16]. Further understanding of regional P/V curves and interpretation of how inflection points can be interpreted, may lead to a better tailoring of ventilation on single patient characteristics.

Conclusion

Pressure-volume curves are a respiratory monitoring technique, readily available at the bedside, that can be performed in paralyzed, mechanically ventilated patients. P/V curve show a sigmoidal shape; variation in compliance along the curve have been physiologically explained in both animal and pathological models. Inflection points of the curve have been interpreted as possible targets for titrating PEEP and plateau pressures during mechanical ventilation, in order to avoid cyclic collapse and/or overdistention of parenchyma during tidal ventilation.

P/V curve study has been extensively applied to ARDS pathophysiology, showing that lower compliance and inhomogeneities in diseased parenchyma is present, further exposing these patients to ventilator-induced lung injury (VILI). Recent evidence suggests that the regional behavior of the P/V curve may differ from global P/V in shape and inflection points, thus highlighting the heterogeneous distribution of pressures along the parenchyma during ventilation.

References

[1] Harris, RS. "Pressure volume curves of the respiratory system." *Respiratory Care,* January 2005, 50 (1) 78-99.

[2] Polese, G., A. Rossi, L. Appendini, G. Brandi, J. H. Bates, and R. Brandolese. "Partitioning of Respiratory Mechanics in Mechanically Ventilated Patients." *Journal of Applied Physiology*. American Physiological Society, December 1, 1991.

[3] Brochard, L., "What is a pressure-volume curve?" *Critical Care.* BioMed Central Ltd, August 10, 2006.

[4] Venegas, José G., R. Scott Harris, and Brett A. Simon. "A Comprehensive Equation for the Pulmonary Pressure-Volume Curve." *Journal of Applied Physiology.* American Physiological Society, January 1, 1998.

[5] Jonson, B., and C. Svantesson. "Elastic Pressure-Volume Curves: What Information Do They Convey?" Thorax. *BMJ*, January 1, 1999.

[6] Gattinoni, Luciano, Antonio Pesenti, Leonello Avalli, Francesca Rossi, and Michela Bombino. "Pressure-Volume Curve of Total Respiratory System in Acute Respiratory Failure: Computed Tomographic Scan Study." *American Review of Respiratory Disease.* American Thoracic Society, August 1987.

[7] Albaiceta, Guillermo M., Francisco Taboada, Diego Parra, Armando Blanco, Dolores Escudero, and Jesús Otero. "Differences in the Deflation Limb of the Pressure-Volume Curves in Acute Respiratory Distress Syndrome from Pulmonary and Extrapulmonary Origin." *Intensive Care Medicine.* Springer Science and Business Media LLC, August 27, 2003.

[8] Hickling, Keith G. "The Pressure–Volume Curve Is Greatly Modified by Recruitment." *American Journal of Respiratory and Critical Care Medicine.* American Thoracic Society, July 1998.

[9] Amato, Marcelo Britto Passos, Carmen Silvia Valente Barbas, Denise Machado Medeiros, Ricardo Borges Magaldi, Guilherme Paula Schettino, Geraldo Lorenzi-Filho, Ronaldo Adib Kairalla, Daniel Deheinzelin, Carlos Munoz, Roselaine Oliveira, Teresa Yae Takagaki, and Carlos Roberto Ribeiro Carvalho, "Effect of a Protective-Ventilation Strategy on Mortality in the Acute Respiratory Distress Syndrome." *New England Journal of Medicine.* Massachusetts Medical Society, February 5, 1998.

[10] Gattinoni, Luciano, and Michael Quintel. "How ARDS Should Be Treated." *Critical Care.* Springer Science and Business Media LLC, April 6, 2016.

[11] Protti, Alessandro, Massimo Cressoni, Alessandro Santini, Thomas Langer, Cristina Mietto, Daniela Febres, Monica Chierichetti, drivi "Lung Stress and Strain during Mechanical Ventilation." *American Journal of Respiratory and Critical Care Medicine.* American Thoracic Society, May 15, 2011.

[12] Terragni, P.P., G.L. Rosboch, A. Lisi, A.G. Viale, and V.M. Ranieri. "How Respiratory System Mechanics May Help in Minimizing Ventilator-Induced Lung Injury in ARDS Patients." *European Respiratory Journal.* European Respiratory Society (ERS), August 1, 2003.

[13] Scaramuzzo, Gaetano, Savino Spadaro, Andreas D. Waldmann, Stephan H. Böhm, Riccardo Ragazzi, Elisabetta Marangoni, Valentina Alvisi, Elena Spinelli, Tommaso Mauri, and Carlo Alberto Volta. "Heterogeneity of Regional Inflection Points from Pressure-Volume Curves Assessed by Electrical Impedance Tomography." *Critical Care.* Springer Science and Business Media LLC, April 16, 2019.

[14] Chen, Lu, Lorenzo Del Sorbo, Domenico Luca Grieco, Orest Shklar, Detajin Junhasavasdikul, Irene Telias, Eddy Fan, and Laurent Brochard. "Airway Closure in Acute Respiratory Distress Syndrome: An Underestimated and Misinterpreted

Phenomenon." *American Journal of Respiratory and Critical Care Medicine.* American Thoracic Society, January 2018.

[15] Massimo Cressoni, Chiara Chiurazzi, Miriam Gotti, Martina Amini, Matteo Brioni, Ilaria Algieri, Antonio Cammaroto, Cristina Rovati, Dario Massari, Caterina Bacile di Castiglione, Klodiana Nikolla, Claudia Montaruli, Marco Lazzerini, Daniele Dondossola, Angelo Colombo, Stefano Gatti, Vincenza Valerio, Nicoletta Gagliano, Eleonora Carlesso, Luciano Gattinoni "Lung Inhomogeneities and Time Course of Ventilator-Induced Mechanical Injuries." Anesthesiology. *Ovid Technologies* (Wolters Kluwer Health), September 1, 2015.

[16] Amato, Marcelo B.P., Maureen O. Meade, Arthur S. Slutsky, Laurent Brochard, Eduardo L.V. Costa, David A. Schoenfeld, Thomas E. Stewart, Matthias Briel, Daniel Talmor, M.P.H., Alain Mercat, Jean-Christophe M. Richard, Carlos R.R. Carvalho, and Roy G. Brower, "Driving Pressure and Survival in the Acute Respiratory Distress Syndrome." *New England Journal of Medicine.* Massachusetts Medical Society, February 19, 2015.

Chapter 21

Non-Invasive Ventilatory Support and Patient Self-Induced Lung Injury: Pathophysiology

Nermin Zerman*, **MD**

Ahi Evran University Training and Research Hospital, Kirsehir, Turkey

Abstract

Respiratory support is an essential component in patients with respiratory failure in whom hypoxemia and/or hypercapnia cannot be controlled with medical treatment. The positive pressure ventilation (PPV) indicated in such a clinical scenario can be applied invasively or noninvasively. The application of non-invasive ventilation (NIV) mitigates the risk of developing complications, especially from intubation. It also reduces the mortality risk associated with invasive mechanical ventilation (IMV).

The oxygenation improvement coupled with lung and diaphragm protection produced by NIV may help to prevent complications. However, in recent years, the phenomenon of patient self-induced lung injury (P-SILI), i.e., the possibility of lung injury induced or worsened by the patient's own inspiratory effort, has emerged. In patients with lung injury leading to an increased inspiratory effort, spontaneous breathing entails the risk of generating high transpulmonary pressure fluctuations and local lung overstrain.

Although no studies have yet demonstrated that a ventilation strategy to limit the risk of P-SILI can improve outcome, the concept of P-SILI is based on sound physiological judgment, the accumulation of clinical observations, and consistent experimental data. Further research, needed to determine the best non-invasive strategy during *de novo* hypoxemic respiratory failure.

* Corresponding Author's Email: nerminzerm@gmail.com.

In: Ventilator Induced Lung Injury in Non-Invasive Ventilatory Support
Editor: Antonio M. Esquinas
ISBN: 979-8-88697-840-7

In this chapter, we discuss the ways to identify the conditions at risk for ventilation-dependent lung injury during NIV in a clinical setting and the extent to which this can help personalize treatment strategies.

Keywords: non-invasive mechanic ventilation (NIV), management, patient self-induced lung injury (P-SILI), prevent, ventilation-induced lung injury (VILI).

Introduction

Mechanical ventilation acts as a life-saving intervention in patients with Acute Respiratory Failure. However, ventilation-induced lung injury (VILI) is a potentially life-threatening complication. VILI is an acute lung injury caused or exacerbated by mechanical ventilation during PPV. It can occur during both IMV and NIV and significantly contributes to the morbidity and mortality of critically ill patients. The impact of VILI on mortality and morbidity is increasingly being recognized worldwide. The concept of injury by mechanical ventilation was introduced in 1744 when John Fothergill expressed the view that after a patient is resuscitated by mouth-to-mouth ventilation, it may be a better option than machine bellows. During the 1952 polio epidemic, researchers documented structural lung damage caused by mechanical ventilation. The ARDSNet trial for VILI was a landmark study that emphasized the importance of low tidal volume ventilation [1].

The predominant mechanisms by which VILI occurs include alveolar hyperplasia (volutrauma), barotrauma, atelectotrauma, and inflammation (biotrauma). Volutrauma refers to lung injury caused by exposure to high tidal volume (VT) that causes alveolar over swelling. Excessive swelling of the lung causes over distension of the small airways and alveoli, resulting in acute edema [2].

Barotrauma refers to lung damage caused by overstretching of the airways and alveoli due to exposure to excessive positive pressure. Atelectrauma depends on ventilation at low lung volumes [3]. Biotrauma results from the release of inflammatory mediators (cytokines and chemokines) secondary to injuries, which are caused by volutrauma, barotrauma, atelectrauma, and sepsis, magnifying the initial damage to the lungs [1].

In addition to these mechanisms for VILI, the concept of P-SILI has emerged in recent years. Exercise-induced lung injury named ‘patient self-induced lung injury (P-SILI) in 2017. According to this concept, during invasive or non-invasive ventilation, the patients might themselves inflict lung injury with a high tidal volume that caused by increased respiratory effort [4].

Conditions in NIV-Acute Hypoxemic Respiratory Failure

Non-invasive respiratory support includes high-flow nasal oxygen (HFNO), NIV, or continuous positive airway pressure (CPAP) delivered through face masks or helmets. NIV is delivered as biphasic positive airway pressure (primarily pressure support ventilation [PSV] = pressure support + PEEP) or CPAP. Both CPAP and PSV-NIV prevent diaphragmatic dysfunction and atrophy associated with spontaneous breathing. They also assist in maintaining the cardiac preload and cardiac output and providing a greater degree of ventilation to the dependent areas of the lung, thus, minimizing the ventilation/perfusion mismatch. They reduce the risk of delirium by maintaining the alertness of the patients and their interaction with the environment. Non-invasive oxygenation strategies preserve the physiological pathways of airway protection (e.g., cough and clearance of secretions). PSV-NIV also reduces the inspiratory effort and work of breathing [5].

However, in patients with lung injury leading to an increased inspiratory effort coupled with a mechanical increase in inspiratory airway pressure, spontaneous breathing entails the risk of generating high transpulmonary pressure fluctuations and local lung overstrain. This further causes additional lung injury (P-SILI), so patients intubated after a trial of non-invasive support are at a higher risk of mortality. Clinical outcome improves when non-invasive support successfully permits to avoid endotracheal intubation.

Conversely, if intubation is required after a failed attempt at non-invasive support, there is an increased risk of mortality due to prolonged exposure of injured lungs to additional damage caused by an increased respiratory effort. Therefore, in patients with hypoxemic respiratory failure need to be consider in selecting patients who will undergo noninvasive ventilation. In mild-to-moderate hypoxemia ($PaO_2/FiO_2 > 150$ mmHg), non-invasive strategies are usually safe and effective and may cause delayed intubation and increased mortality in a considerable proportion of moderate-to-severe ($PaO_2/FiO_2 \leq 150$ mmHg) cases [6].

NIV is a process by which mechanical ventilation can be applied without needing intubation. Generally, hypoxemic respiratory failure is more difficult to treat with NIV than hypercapnic respiratory failure. NIV is increasingly used to aid spontaneous breathing during acute hypoxic de novo respiratory failure (AHRF), although its potential therapeutic effect is controversial. Previous data suggest that, regardless of the severity of the respiratory failure, the use of NIV in patients with ARDS is associated with higher mortality in the event of failure. Therefore, the use of NIV requires caution due to an increase in the mortality rate due to delayed endotracheal intubation [7].

The success of NIV also depends on the initial severity of the disease. In most studies, the disease severity was determined by APACHE II score and Simplified Acute Physiology Score (SAPS II) score. There are diverse studies that have reported an increase in these scores being associated with NIV failure. In a multicenter, prospective study by Antonelli et al., including 1809 patients, the initial SAPS II score, presence of comorbidity, pH at baseline and at the end of the first hour, PaO_2/FIO_2 ratio were found to be independent risk factors for hospital mortality for NIV success. According to this study, patients with multiple comorbidities, higher disease severity, and no improvement in arterial blood gas values at the end of the first hour do not benefit from NIV [8].

There are multiple complementary mechanisms underlying additional lung injury due to increased respiratory efforts during NIV. Spontaneous breathing has diverse mechanisms of injury:

1) An increase in the respiratory impulse leads to an increase in the patient's respiratory efforts, tidal volume, and transpulmonary pressure (PL) above safe limits. Spontaneous breathing in the ventilator reduces pleural pressure and increases transpulmonary pressure, and therefore, increases tidal volume for the same mechanical properties of the lung. This pause increases the likelihood of barotrauma during pressure-targeted ventilation. Along with the underlying lung damage, these changes can be significantly detrimental.
2) In conditions with a lung injury, spontaneous effort leads to a pendulum phenomenon (that is, gas exchange occurs from non-dependent areas to dependent areas due to differential changes in pleural pressure). In undamaged lungs, spontaneous effort leads to a uniform change in pleural pressure throughout inspiration, resulting in a uniform change in transpulmonary pressure. However, in damaged lungs, the spontaneous effort results in a higher and earlier negative pleural pressure in the dependent areas compared to non-dependent areas. This causes the air to become dependent on non-dependent areas in the early phase of inspiration. The swelling from

such prolapses can cause a significant tidal uptake of dependent regions, and the collapsed and consolidated lung creates parenchymal mechanical heterogeneities in the damaged lung, increasing the risk of volutrauma through regional stress amplification.

3) An overall negative intrathoracic pressure results from the negative pleural pressure created due to spontaneous exertion. This increases the venous return and lung perfusion leading to high intravascular pressure. During ventilation, spontaneous effort causes a decrease in airway pressure and an increase in transvascular pressure. This increases the tendency of forming pulmonary edema.
4) Spontaneous effort can also worsen the patient-ventilator mismatch. Conducted VT and transpulmonary pressure may be higher, especially in the case of double or reverse triggering. Thus, despite lung-sparing strategies, it may worsen lung injury leading to inferior outcomes.
5) Diaphragm injury occurs if the respiratory impulse causes severe spontaneous respiratory efforts [3,9].
6) Patient intolerance or air leaks during NIV can result in intermittent mask removal and an increase in the respiratory drive, promoting patient-ventilator mismatch [10].

The increased respiratory drive may also be caused by multiple mechanisms such as gas exchange and deterioration in respiratory mechanics, metabolic acidosis, inflammation, fever, and agitation. The intense inspiratory effort, with or without additional mechanical support, results in high tidal volumes and tachypnea [6].

Diagnosis of P-SILI

Safe spontaneous breathing is a challenge as it should aim to minimize the volume and transpulmonary pressure (PL) to avoid P-SILI, while at the same time providing an appropriate level of patient respiratory effort to prevent diaphragmatic atrophy. Close monitoring of respiration is the key. There are no clear diagnostic criteria for P-SILI. The electrical activity of the diaphragm (EAdi) represents the "closest" proxy of the neural respiratory system available in clinical practice. Eadi recorded using a multi-lead esophageal catheter. The ratio of tidal volume (Vt) to EAdi represents the near ventilation efficiency of the diaphragm.

An esophageal catheter can help in a reliable assessment of respiratory effort by recording the esophageal pressure (Pes) signal as an estimation of pleural pressure. Esophageal manometry used for clinical and research purposes to measure pleural pressures, predict chest wall mechanics, isolate chest wall effects, and determine expanding pressures in the lungs. In addition, pressure-based indices developed by respiratory muscles, such as respiratory effort esophageal pressure fluctuations (ΔPes), and respiratory muscle pressure (Pmus), provide reliable quantification of inspiratory effort determined by the neural respiratory impulse. Negative airway pressure created by occlusion during the first 0.1 s of an inspiration, known as P 0.1, commonly used as an index of respiratory impulse. In healthy subjects P 0.1, ranges from 0.5 to 1.5 cmH_2O. P0.1 values consistently above 3–4 cmH_2O indicate high neural respiratory impulse and high work of breathing [10].

A diaphragm ultrasound is used to evaluate patient-ventilator interactions and measure the thickening fraction (TFdi) associated with inspiratory effort. A TF of less than .15% is a sign of over-help, while a TF of over 30% to 40% is a sign of under-aid [4].

Therapeutic Interventions

Extreme caution must be exercised to avoid the high inspiratory effort to limit VILI and P-SILI in acute respiratory failure. Three approaches have proposed to minimize P-SILI:

1) *Limitation of tidal volume.* Carteaux *et al.,* demonstrated that an exhaled Vt greater than 9.5 mL/kg during NIV is an independent risk factor for NIV failure [11,12]. Vt is not usually measured during NIV, and the clinical response inferred by a decrease in respiratory effort. A high respiratory effort implies high tidal volume, and the persistence of such high effort has been hypothesized to cause self-inflicted lung injury [3].
2) *PEEP implementation.* Implementation of high PEEP levels is also promising for the prevention of P-SILI. The effectiveness of PEEP in reducing P-SILI explained by fewer atelectatic areas and peripheral airway collapse, a more homogeneous distribution of inspiratory stress, reduced regional overstrain in dependent areas, and reduced pressures generated by spontaneous efforts. PEEP improves gas exchange, which can potentially reduce the respiratory drive [11]. In

addition, PEEP exerts a direct mechanical effect on the diaphragm by changing the force-length relationship of the muscle fibers. Recently, it has been determined that administration of moderate to elevated levels of PEEP (10–15 cmH_2O) during spontaneous breathing and ARDS improves ventilation uniformity and prevents "*pendelluf* "phenomena through a more even distribution of negative inspiratory pressure throughout the lung tissue. For these reasons, strategies of administrating higher levels of PEEP through non-invasive support may contribute to reduced respiratory drive [6].

3) *Reduction of spontaneous effort.* All these strategies must combine with appropriate sedation and metabolic control. Firstly, non-respiratory factors that may increase the respiratory drive, such as pain, mask intolerance, metabolic acidosis, and fever must be corrected. The neuropsychiatric component of the respiratory drive (delirium, fear) could be addressed via appropriately established drug or non-drug concepts. Pharmacological agents can be used to reduce respiratory drive. Propofol and benzodiazepines have been shown to reduce respiratory effort. Opioids reduce the respiratory rate with mixed effects on Vt and inspiratory effort but may increase the risk of apnea. Measures with side effects such as neuromuscular blockade or deep analgesia only if the probability of P SILI is extremely high [6].

Different interfaces are available for NIV: The preferred interfaces are full face masks and helmets. Helmet-type masks consist of a transparent cap that covers the patient's entire head with a soft-collar neck seal. Due to the lack of contact with the face and the integrity of the seal on the neck, helmets are better accepted. It can allow positive airway pressures (PEEP 8–12 cmH_2O) to increase as it creates less air leakage compared to a face mask. NIV delivered via a helmet can potentially provide additional protection against P-SILI [13].

If there is an impending or significant P-SILI despite the exhaustion of the indicated measures, IMV should be applied by stopping spontaneous breathing by deepening analgesic sedation and, if necessary, completing neuromuscular blockade [14].

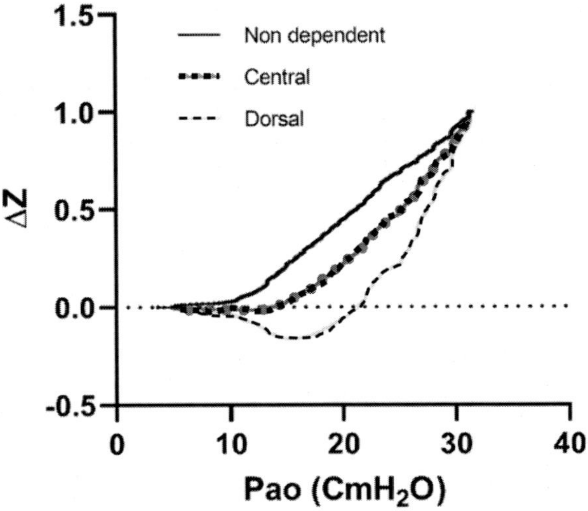

ΔZ= variation of impedance; Pao= airway opening pressure. The 3 curves represent the behavior of 3 different lung regions, i.e., the non-dependent (black), central (dark grey) and dependent lung (light grey). It can be noted how the lower inflection point moves to higher values of pressure going from the non-dependent to the dependent lung region.

Figure 1. Example of EIT derived regional pressure volume curves in an ARDS patient.

Conclusion

In recent years, the concept of P-SILI has emerged as the cause of VILI. Caution must be in selecting patients who will undergo NIV in patients with hypoxemic respiratory failure. In mild to moderate hypoxemia (PaO_2/FiO_2 > 150 mmHg), NIV may be a safe and effective option. It recommended to keep the Vt low and apply high PEEP to minimize P-SILI. In addition, the use of a helmet-type mask should be recommended during NIV. Apart from these measures, causes of hyperventilation such as metabolic acidosis, pain, agitation, and fever were evaluated and controlled. Endotracheal intubation needs to be planned if P-SILI cannot be prevented despite all these precautions.

Future research should focus specifically on monitoring P-SILI and better defining the preventive strategy during both invasive and non-invasive ventilation supports.

References

[1] Beitler J R, Malhotra A, Thompson BT. Ventilator-induced Lung Injury. *Clin. Chest. Med.* 2016 Dec;37(4):633–646. doi: 10.1016/j.ccm.2016.07.004. Epub 2016 Oct 14. PMID: 27842744; PMCID: PMC5131805.

[2] Faridy E E, Permutt S, Riley R L. Effect of ventilation on surface forces in excised dogs' lungs. *J. Appl. Physiol.* 1966 Sep;21(5):1453–62. doi: 10.1152/jappl.1966.21.5.1453. PMID: 5923215.

[3] Katira B H. Ventilator-Induced Lung Injury: Classic and Novel Concepts. *Respir. Care.* 2019 Jun;64(6):629–637. doi: 10.4187/respcare.07055. PMID: 31110032.

[4] Carteaux G, Parfait, M, Combet, M, Haudebourg, A-F, Tuffet, S, Dessap AM. A. Patient-Self Inflicted Lung Injury: A Practical Review. *J. Clin. Med.* 2021 Jun 21;10(12): 2738. doi: 10.3390/jcm10122738. PMID: 34205783; PMCID: PMC 8234933.

[5] M Antonelli· G Conti, M Rocco, M Bufi, R A De Blasi, G Vivino, A Gasparetto, G U Meduri. A comparison of non-invasive positive-pressure ventilation and conventional mechanical ventilation in patients with acute respiratory failure. *N. Engl. J. Med.* 1998 Aug 13;339(7):429–35. doi: 10.1056/NEJM199808133390703. PMID: 9700176.

[6] Domenico Luca Grieco· Salvatore Maurizio Maggiore· Oriol Roca· Elena Spinelli· Bhakti K Patel· Arnaud W Thille, Carmen Sílvia V Barbas· Marina Garcia de Acilu· Salvatore Lucio Cutuli· Filippo Bongiovanni· Marcelo Amato· Jean-Pierre Frat· Tommaso Mauri· John P Kress· Jordi Mancebo· Massimo Antonelli. Non-invasive ventilatory support and high-flow nasal oxygen as first-line treatment of acute hypoxemic respiratory failure and ARDS. *Intensive Care Med.* 2021 47, 851–866 (2021). https://doi.org/10.1007/s00134–021–06459–2.

[7] Roberto Tonelli· Riccardo Fantini· Luca Tabbì· Ivana Castaniere, Lara Pisani· Maria Rosaria Pellegrino· Giovanni Della Casa· Roberto D'Amico, Massimo Girardis· Stefano Nava· Enrico M Clini· Alessandro Marchioni. Early Inspiratory Effort Assessment by Esophageal Manometry Predicts Noninvasive Ventilation Outcome in *De Novo* Respiratory Failure. A Pilot Study. *Am. J. Respir. Crit. Care Med.* 2020 Aug 15;202(4):558–567. doi: 10.1164/rccm.201912–2512OC. PMID: 32325004; PMCID: PMC7427381.

[8] M Antonelli· G Conti, M L Moro, A Esquinas, G Gonzalez-Diaz, M Confalonieri, P Pelaia, T Principi, C Gregoretti, F Beltrame, M A Pennisi, A Arcangeli, R Proietti, M Passariello, G U Meduri. Predictors of failure of non-invasive positive pressure ventilation in patients with acute hypoxemic respiratory failure: a multicenter study. *Intensive Care Med.* 2001;27:1718–28.

[9] Michele Bertoni· Savino Spadaro· Ewan C Goligher. Monitoring Patient Respiratory Effort During Mechanical Ventilation: Lung and Diaphragm-Protective Ventilation. *Crit Care* 24, 106 (2020). https://doi.org/10.1186/s13054–020–2777-y.

[10] Elena Spinelli· Tommaso Mauri· Jeremy R Beitler· Antonio Pesenti· Daniel Brodie. Respiratory drive in the acute respiratory distress syndrome: pathophysiology, monitoring, and therapeutic interventions. *Intensive Care Med.* 2020 Apr;46(4): 606–618.

[11] Denise Battaglini· Chiara Robba· Lorenzo Ball· Pedro L Silva· Fernanda F Cruz· Paolo Pelosi· Patricia R M Rocco. Non-invasive respiratory support, and patient self-inflicted lung injury in COVID-19: a narrative review. *Br. J. Anaesth.* 2021 Sep;127(3):353–364. doi: 10.1016/j.bja.2021.05.024.

[12] Guillaume Carteaux· Teresa Millán-Guilarte, Nicolas De Prost, Keyvan Razazi, Shariq Abid, Arnaud W Thille, Frédérique Schortgen, Laurent Brochard, Christian Brun-Buisson, Armand Mekontso Dessap . "Failure of non-invasive ventilation for de novo acute hypoxemic respiratory failure: role of tidal volume." *Critical Care Medicine* 44.2 (2016): 282–290.

[13] Domenico L Grieco· Luca S Menga, Davide Eleuteri, Massimo Antonelli. Patient self-inflicted lung injury: implications for acute hypoxemic respiratory failure and ARDS patients on non-invasive support. Minerva *Anesthesiology.* 2019 Sep;85(9): 1014–1023. doi: 10.23736/S0375–9393.19.13418–9. Epub 2019 Mar 12. PMID: 30871304.

[14] Benjamin Neetz· Thomas Flohr· Felix J F Herth· Michael M Müller. Patient self-inflicted lung injury" (P-SILI) : Von der Pathophysiologie zur klinischen Evaluation mit differenziertem Management [*Patient self-inflicted lung injury (P-SILI) : From pathophysiology to clinical evaluation with differentiated management*]. *Med. Klin. Intensivmed Notfmed.* 2021 Oct;116(7):614–623. German. doi: 10.1007/s00063–021–00823–2. Epub 2021 May 7. PMID: 33961061; PMCID: PMC8103432.

Index

A

L

M

N

O

T

Editor's Contact Information

Antonio M. Esquinas, M.D, Ph.D, FCCP,
International Fellow AARC
Intensive Care Unit,
Hospital Morales Meseguer, Murcia, Spain
antmesquinas@gmail.com